SpringerBriefs in Computer Science

More information about this series at http://www.springer.com/series/10028

Honggang Wang · Md Shaad Mahmud
Hua Fang · Chonggang Wang

Wireless Health

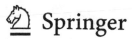 Springer

Honggang Wang
Department of Electrical and Computer
    Engineering
University of Massachusetts Dartmouth
Dartmouth
MA
USA

Md Shaad Mahmud
Department of Electrical and Computer
    Engineering
University of Massachusetts Dartmouth
Dartmouth
MA
USA

Hua Fang
Department of Quantitative
    Health Sciences
University of Massachusetts Medical
    School
Worcester
MA
USA

Chonggang Wang
InterDigital Communications
King of Prussia
USA

ISSN 2191-5768   ISSN 2191-5776   (electronic)
SpringerBriefs in Computer Science
ISBN 978-3-319-47945-3   ISBN 978-3-319-47946-0   (eBook)
DOI 10.1007/978-3-319-47946-0

Library of Congress Control Number: 2016955067

Printed on acid-free paper

This Springer imprint is published by Springer Nature
The registered company is Springer International Publishing AG
The registered company address is: Gewerbestrasse 11, 6330 Cham, Switzerland

Preface

This concise book provides a candid assessment and practical knowledge about the current technological advancements of the wireless healthcare system. The text presents the competencies of modeling e-health framework, medical wireless body sensor networks, communication technologies for mobile health, nanotechnology innovations in medicine, security issues for medical records, personalized services in healthcare applications, and Big Data for wireless health.

This book covers multiple research perspectives in order to address the strong need for interdisciplinary research in the area of wireless health, such as the interactive research among biomedical sensor technology, intelligent textiles and advanced wireless network technology. The interactions involve experts from multidisciplinary fields including medical, information technology and computing fields. Designed as a study tool for graduate students, researchers, and medical professionals, this book is also valuable for business managers, entrepreneurs, and investors within the medical and healthcare industries. It is useful for anyone who cares about the future opportunities in healthcare systems.

We are deeply indebted to colleagues and students who have read this material and given us valuable suggestions for improving the presentation. Especially, there are many suggestions from researchers who participate in IEEE/ACM conference on connected health: Applications, Systems and Engineering Technologies (CHASE) co-founded by Weisong Shi and one of authors Honggang Wang. We owe a special debt of gratitude to Sherman Shen from University of waterloo who initiated this book opportunity, read the original manuscript in detail and gave us valuable advices. We also want to thank Susan Lagerstrom-Fife and Jennifer Malat from Springer for their great support.

We present this book with a hope that more and more readers could follow up the direction of wireless health in the future.

Dartmouth, USA   Honggang Wang
Dartmouth, USA   Md Shaad Mahmud
Worcester, USA   Hua Fang
King of Prussia, USA   Chonggang Wang

Acknowledgment

We would like to acknowledge the in part the support from by This work was supported in part by the National Science Foundation (NSF) within the Division of Information and Intelligent Systems under Grant 1401711, in part by NSF within the Division of Electrical, Communications and Cyber Systems under Grant 1407882, in part by the National Institute of Health (NIH) within the National Center for Advancing Translational Sciences under Grant 5UL1TR000161-04, and in part by NIH and the National Institute on Drug Abuse under Grant 1R01DA033323-01.

Contents

Chapter 1
Introduction

1.1 Background

The rapid growth of wireless communication and networks makes the devices and people connected and have been significantly shaping people life to a new model. It also has fostered many new applications. Among them, wireless health is one of the most critical technologies and has brought huge number of exciting wireless mobile health applications, which are improving human wellbeing and reducing the increasing worldwide healthcare cost. Wireless health is defined as the technology that relies on wireless communication infrastructure to monitor and diagnose people's healthcare anytime and anywhere, and thus improve people's healthcare. There are several trends in recent years regarding the growth of wireless health:

- Personalized telemedicine: The medicine will be customized for each individual based on each user's needs;
- The transformation from reactive care to proactive and preventive care;
- Internet of Things (IoT) helps the growth of wireless health. Healthcare monitoring using the sensors and wireless communication can be realized anywhere and anytime.
- Cloud and real time big data analytics provide tools for the real time or near real time healthcare data analysis and provide healthcare decision and suggestions.

At the same time, wireless communications and networks still keeps growing. For example, 5G wireless technologies will enable much larger volume data exchange in real time and enable many wireless applications. Future internet will have more flexible architecture and can accommodate the demands of many applications as needed. A new term called "Internet+" is becoming popular especially in China, which has tremendous growth on the internet applications. With more and more understanding the relationships between the digital information and healthcare, a new term called smart and connected health also emerge in recent years. With the

© The Author(s) 2016
H. Wang et al., *Wireless Health*, SpringerBriefs in Computer Science,
DOI 10.1007/978-3-319-47946-0_1

help of the wireless networks and internet, more and more devices and people are connected through them. Physiological signal from human beings' body are collected and sent to central servers or remote cloud and will be analyzed.

On the other hand, Wearable technology, as major part of wireless health, perhaps the most prolific topic in technological industries. From activity-tracking fitness bands of a wrist watch to Google Glass and Oculus Rift, big names with bigger visions are involved in the once-niche technology. You probably wouldn't have guessed that the technology would be so much accessible compare to 60s, where the first attempt of wearable devices was introduced to cheat in casinos. Throughout the 1960s–70s there were couple wearable devices to count cards and improve the odds at the roulette table. In the following, especially, we introduce the timeline of wearable technologies for the past 10 years, from the Nike Kit to Apple watch.

The Nike+iPod Sports Kit was released in mid-2006. This device can track your activity by counting and recording the number of steps and pace of a walk or run. The IPhone has a separate application to connect the device with the Nike+iPod, which also can communicate with the Nike+ Sport band. These devices can log all the steps and distance travelled by the user.

In 2010, Nike has released another product Nike+ Running App, which uses information of the mobile accelerometer and GPS to step counter and location. The iPhone 1st generation was released in 2007 by Steve Jobs at the Macworld convention. It was the first of its capacitive based touch pad with quad-band GSM cellular connectivity with GPRS and EDGE support for data transfer. In 2008, Apple announced its updated version, iPhone 3G.

Fitbit was founded by James Park and Eric Friedman. It was first released in 2008, Park mentioned that they had to go under 7 times due to manufacturing faultiness. Fitbit was initially and activity tracker with wireless capability, it can measure and store vital information such as number of steps walked, heart rate, quality of sleep, steps climbed, and other personal metrics. Fitbit tracker is its first edition of all the releases.

Jawbone, a wearable device manufacturing company was founded by Alexander Asseily and Hosain Rahman. Initially, the name of the company was Aliph where they were working together on noise cancellation for DARPA. During the span of 2009–2011 they introduced different Bluetooth headsets and finally in 2011 by releasing Jawbone ERA they also rebranded the company to "Jawbone".

Nike FuelBand is an activity tracker which worn on the wrist, also work with Android and IOS platform. FuelBand allows its users to track their daily activity, number of steps, and amount of calorie burned. The information from the FuelBand is connected to Nike+ community and server, allowing wearers to set their own fitness goals, monitor their progress, and compare themselves to others part of the community. Nike+ relies on the gamification of fitness activities turning all tracked movement into NikeFuel points, which can unlock achievements, can be shared with friends, or can be used to engage others in competition.

The Nissan Nismo watch was released in 2013, it allows car drivers to monitor the efficiency of the vehicle. The wrist watch displays the car speed, fuel consumption and lock and unlock the doors. It can also perform personal activity monitor with heart rate monitor. It also enables to interest you with the social media such as Facebook, Twitter and instagram and keeps you updated with your recent posts.

Misfit's Shine is a wearable device released in 2013, and it allows the wearer to monitor sleep and track movements to calculate different level of metrics like sleep count, calorie counter and light or deep sleep monitor. It works with IOS, Android and windows platform.

Google Glass is an optical head-mounted display that is designed in the shape of a pair of eyeglasses. Google glass was developed by Google X team and first introduced in 2013. Later in 2014, they started to sell it commercially, but was criticized due to safety and security issues.

Wristwatches evolved with time and have adopted new technologies to do more than just displaying time and date. Apple watch and Samsung watch are quite similar in terms of performance and accessibility. It allows you to make calls, access the Internet, activity monitor, personal health tracker and more.

Recently a new era of virtual reality devices has been introduced to the world of wearable devices. The "Oculus Rift", consists of built in headphones, motion sensor and display lets the user to step in virtual worlds like games, movies (Oculus, n.d.). What is clear is that, based on the history of wearable technology, devices that move the masses are far and between. The successes that do make it, however, can change the world and generate charts-topping returns.

Therefore, we will give an overview of wireless network and sensor technology in the following sections.

1.2   Overview of Wireless Network and Sensor Technology

The term sensor refers to a device that transform the physical signal to an electrical signal. Especially in the case of biomedical devices the use of sensors has moved from scientific research to daily life application—socializing, fitness, health monitoring, sports, and military. The reason behind this migration is due to the enhancement of the sensor and integration with the "Wireless Health". For biological information the signals are so much unpredictable and highly susceptible to environmental and physiological noises/art effects. The sensor is the media by which we quantize the physical world to electrical signal. In recent years there has been a great enhancement in sensor manufacturing and making them cost effective. In addition to this, researchers combine these intelligent sensors with miniature microprocessor for scientific, industrial and consumer applications. Wireless network has been introduced for remote monitoring and increasing comfortless of the targeted users. Wireless part is necessary to transmit and receive information's from sensor nodes to the central unit.

1.3 Overview of Smart and Connected Health

Smart and connected health involves sensing, communications and smart system such as decision support system. Wireless body sensor network is a fundamental infrastructure of smart and connected health. Enabling future smart and connected health requires the integration of these technologies from all three aspects. There are other similar terms related to smart and connected health such as mobile health, e-health. A typical smart and connected health system is automatic drug delivery for diabetes person, where glucose sensors collect the glucose level in the blood and wirelessly transmit the signal to pump that is deployed on the same body. The pump will inject insulin to the blood according to the received glucose level. This is a loop medical cyber physical system which involves the sensing, wireless communications and intelligent decision. There are many challenges for building up smart and connected health system. The first major challenge is the sensor design. For example, the sensor must be small size (e.g., wearable), power efficient. On the other side, the software on the sensor must lightweight due to the limited computing resources. The second major challenge is the communication efficiency. Especially, the communication is the dominator factor for the energy consumption. Considering limited energy resource (e.g., battery support), the communication protocol must also be designed with energy efficiency. The protocol design involves multiple layers. Although IEEE.802.16 has a standard for wireless body area networks. However, the standard has not been widely adopted. The third challenge is about the smart and intelligent techniques. It is critical to discover the key information from the collected signal by sensors. In some applications, a real-time data analytic is required, which poses challenge in the design of computational efficient algorithms.

Clearly, it's not easy to manage all these data from thousands of nodes collecting information. Some significant questions are raised: for example, how can we manipulate, process, store and maintain the quality of the services? Not to mention, keeping all the personal and health information secure at the same time. Answers to these questions will be complex and depends on how we organize and finance health organizations. Nevertheless, a part of the solution may be solved by how and to what extent we take benefit of recent advances in modern electronics and technology or related fields. Presently, there are technologies that hold great promise to expand the capabilities of the healthcare system, extending its range into the community, improving diagnostics and monitoring, and maximizing the independence and participation of individuals (Cornelius, 2014). Therefore, we will be focusing on remote monitoring systems based on wearable technology. We chose to focus on these technologies due to the fact that current developments in wearable sensor technology have led to a number of thrilling clinical applications.

Wearable sensors can be used to diagnose, as well as process real time life threatening conditions. Their current capabilities include physiological and biochemical sensing, as well as motion sensing. It might be difficult to measure the problems which may be solved by using wearable technology. Monitoring health in real time could improve in both diagnosis and ongoing treatment of a vast number of individuals with neurological, cardiovascular and respiratory diseases such as seizures, hypertension, dysthymias, and asthma. Sensors like motion and posture could solve falls prevention and maximize the efficiency of individual's and community contribution. Wireless health monitoring systems have the potential to minimize problematic patient access issues. Approximately 20 % of those in the US live in rural areas, on the other hand only 9 % of the medical doctor work in rural areas. These numbers can get worse over time. There is a huge background of literature that describes the differences in care faced by rural residents. Compared to people living in urban areas, people living in rural areas travel 2 or 3 times further to see a medical doctor, which takes more time, cost and unreliable for patients with severe health conditions. Wearable sensors and remote monitoring systems have the potential to extend the reach of specialists in urban areas to rural areas and decrease these disparities.

A conceptual representation of a wearable system for wireless health monitoring includes sensing, communications and decision support and data processing. Wearable sensors are capable of gathering physiological data which enable to monitor patients continuously. Sensors are deployed according to the clinical application of interest. Wearable sensors to monitor vital signs could be deployed in monitoring patients with heart conditions or patients with chronic obstructive pulmonary disease. Motion sensors with actual movement and posture detection can be used to monitor the effectiveness of home-based rehabilitation interventions in stroke survivors or assistance of disabled people. These sensor nodes equipped with wireless module which relied on a sensor such as mobile phone or access point and store the information to cloud via internet for post processing. In case of emergency, stored data can be retrieved instantly for the medical history of the patient, also real time monitoring can trigger an alarm message to emergency service center to provide immediate assistance. Patients can also use wearable sensors as a reminder of taking medicines, and family members and medical persons are notified in case of an emergency as well as in other situations, for instance, taking the patient in a periodic medication. Medical personnel can monitor the patient's status from a remote place and can be informed in case a medical decision has to be made.

The integration of wearable sensors into the health care system will certainly bring numerous advantages and this will be a seamless transformation with our current health care practices. For example, currently we use wires, patches and adhesive electrodes for monitoring the patient's vital signs, whereas with technological advancement we are tending from wired to wireless. Quality of life of patient has been improving because with wireless module they do not have to lie on the bed for days or see the doctor every other day. Continuous monitoring can be done with wireless sensor network, while the patient is moving and without hampering any daily activities at home or work. Also, instantaneous suggestion regarding health condition can be provided with diagnosis and response can be made promptly. In addition to that, the medical doctors do not have to take care of the patients continuously and therefore will minimize the time and pressure on the overall healthcare system.

Despite all the above mentioned potential advantages, there are still few significant challenges which wearable sensor is suffering from. These challenges include power consumption, miniaturization and last but not least social stigma with use of wearable sensor for home based clinical monitoring. In later sections we will be describing wearable sensor technologies that are essential components of systems to monitor patients in the home and community settings.

Daily Activity Trackers: As the name states, it is a device for tracking your fitness related information for instance distance acquired by walk or run, number calories burnt, quality of the slip, heart rate and respiration. Activity tracker also known as a fitness band or smart watch. Some of the smart watch also performs as a mobile host, through that you can make calls, text and perform hand gestures. Nowadays, activity trackers have been widely used in medical sciences, sports and security. The built sensor can also detect abnormal or unforeseen situation, it also can diagnose and predict through this tracker. This has transformed health care system an easy accessible platform by allowing continuous monitoring of patients without hospitalization.

Activity tracker, looks quite cool and fashionable, but most importantly, it has increased awareness among wearers.

Smart Eyewear: Smart eyewear is a lot look like a pair of eyeglasses with wearable headset, built in display and motion sensor. Google Glass is one of the popular smart eyewear that has been released so far. Initially, it was released at a price of USD 1500 but could not stay for a long in the market because it lacks security and safety features. It has a voice-controlled Android device that displays information directly in the user's field of vision, something that you might have seen in movies like Terminator. Google Glass provides an augmented reality experience by mixing different features like audio, video and motion.

After January, 2015 Google has stopped making Google Glass. However, they mentioned it will be still in the development process to overcome all the drawbacks.

Smart T-shirt: Smart T-shirt or textile is a wearable technology that can monitor and store information's like person's movement, track activity and vital signs. It transmits these data to sensor hub or mobile phone where users can interact and infer their health condition. Also wearer can track their fitness without wearing anything else besides the smart textile.

It can be categorized as two major parts: aesthetic and performance enhancing. Aesthetic smart textile include everything from fabrics that has light emitting diodes to fabrics which can change color on different environmental conditions. Some of these fabrics gather energy from the environment by harnessing vibrations, sound or heat.

Smart Shoe: Smart Shoe is a wearable device, where sensors are placed into shoes pair. It navigates wearer without looking at the application in mobile phone. It connects with the phone through Bluetooth and it vibrates as an alert signal to take the right/left to reach the destination. Smart shoe also has a small buzzer which triggers at the same time when it vibrates. Once the route has been selected, the user need not keep glancing at a smartphone screen.

Wearable Technology has been one of the hottest trends in recent time. There has been a lot of research studies, hence products like Google Glass, Apple watch, Samsung smartwatch, etc. are out there in the market. Many developments are going on, and products are launched every day and we hope to see lots of innovative wearable devices in near future!

1.4 Aim of This Brief

The aim of this brief is to offer an overview of wireless health, including both system design, data analytics and applications. For example, how to design wireless link for body sensor network to perform efficiently without hampering the natural activity of the user. We will also conduct the survey on recent development of different sensors, commercially and non-commercially available. This brief is to provide transformative knowledge for students, researchers, scholars, engineers, medical professionals whose job are to understand/select/design sensors for biomedical devices.

References

Cornelius, C. (2014). A wearable system that knows who wears it. In *Proceedings of the 12th Annual International Conference on Mobile Systems, Applications, and Services* (pp. 55–67). Bretton Woods, New Hampshire, USA: ACM.

Oculus. (n.d.). Retrieved from Oculus https://www.oculus.com/.

Chapter 2
Wireless Health Systems

2.1 Systems

Body Sensor Network can help people by providing healthcare information such as monitoring health, tracking activity, improvement of lifestyle, memory enhancement, and suggestions based on these information. Also it can establish instant communication between healthcare providers in case of emergency. Through BSN it is also possible to acquire remote monitoring without hampering patients' natural movements, hence improvement of lifestyle. Although the present systems allow continuous monitoring but it was wired and consists of bulky devices. But now, with wireless sensor network there is no physical cable connection between sensors and the hubs. However, it is required to be within a certain distance to the central to hub to establish communication. Most of the cases, the wireless connection is made through cellular network, 3G/4G networks or wireless LAN. But the coverage of these network infrastructure is limited and most importantly it can be done with small Bluetooth and any IoT enabled sensors. With the consideration of this, it is better to use BLE, Wi-Fi or ad hoc wireless network for short range communication.

In this section, we will discuss the sensor system, its architecture and how to design and deploy wireless sensor network for health monitoring. Wearable devices allow an individual to monitor his/her health continuously and track any changes of user's vital signs and feedback to maintain a healthy lifestyle. Patients can store and check their health information as a part of diagnostic procedure, and can be supervised in an emergency case or before any surgical procedures. Long term and continuous monitoring have other benefits such as tracking variation of circadian can be a good indicator of cardiac patients.

© The Author(s) 2016
H. Wang et al., *Wireless Health*, SpringerBriefs in Computer Science,
DOI 10.1007/978-3-319-47946-0_2

2.1.1 Sensor Systems

A sensor system can generally be defined as a network of nodes that sense and control the environment, enabling interaction between environment, person or computers. In case of WSN, a large number of sensor nodes, hubs and clients are deployed for health monitoring. Sensor nodes sense and collect data along with other sensors and transmit data by multiple hopping. Multiple hopping sends the data through different nodes to get to the central gateway, and lastly reach the central node to connect to the internet or satellite. Although, user can manage the configuration with WSN management, including publishing data to collection and monitoring data.

Recently, the cost of WSN equipment's has dropped drastically and also it is getting small in size. The application of WSN are not limited to military and industrial fields, application for wearable devices are gradually expanding. Meanwhile, standards for WSN technology has been well improved, such as Bluetooth low energy (BLE), Zigbee and Wi-Fi for short distance commination. The sensor node is one of the major parts of the WSN system. The hardware of the sensor node consists of four modules: sensor, power module which includes power management and charging control system, wireless transceiver and a microcontroller. However, with technological advancement there is wireless microcontroller such as RFduino, Simblee, CC2500, etc. These are BLE enabled microcontrollers, which require less space and low energy to transmit data. The sensor is the core of the WSN and provides the status of the environmental changes like ambient, temperature, vibration and chemical signals. Also it transfers these data to microcontroller to quantify. Microcontroller receives the information and converts it into digital format, also process accordingly. The wireless transceiver then transfers the data to central hub or through multiple nodes. For every sensor node it is important to achieve the moisturize size without compromising power.

The miniaturization technology of WSN nodes based on microelectromechanical systems (MEMS) has made remarkable progress in recent years. The core technology of MEMS is to realize the Combination of microelectronics technology, micromachining technology and the packaging technology. Different levels of 2D and 3D micro sensitive structures can be produced based on microelectronics and micro-machining technology, which can be the miniature sensing elements. These miniature sensing elements, associated power supply and signal conditioning circuits can be integrated and packaged as a miniature MEMS sensor. In recent days, there are many types of miniature MEMS sensors in the market which can be used to measure vital signs, velocity, pressure, strain, stress, light, heat, pH, etc. In year 2003, University of California Berkley first introduced a WSN sensor node with micro sensor, the actual size was 2.8 mm by 2.1 mm.

To perform all these tasks, nodes need power, besides traditional battery, an energy harvesting module can be used. These systems are inexpensive, small and product enough energy to run the whole system for several days. However, life time of these modules depends on the system architecture. There are some devices in the market which have already used energy acquisition. For example, German company EnOcean produces energy harvesting module from light, vibration and temperature. For health monitoring nodes, different kind of piezoelectric energy harvesting module has been seen in the market. A British company named Perpetuum offers a module that can convert mechanical vibration to electrical energy. For these sensor nodes the energy of vibration made by your fingers knocking the desk can support the sensor node sending 2 kB data to 100 m away every 60 second.

2.1.2 Network Infrastructure

WSNs are pivotal parts of the multilayer system. Each sensor node can sense, process, and transmit the data to different node or to central hub. Most of the time, nodes are integrated with multiple sensors to measure physiological sensor. For example, electrocardiogram sensor (ECG) can be used for monitoring heart activity, an electromyogram sensor (EMG) for monitoring muscle activity, an electroencephalogram sensor (EEG) for monitoring brain electrical activity, a blood pressure sensor for monitoring blood pressure, a pressure sensor for monitoring movement, and a breathing sensor for monitoring respiration; and motion sensors can be used to discriminate the user's status and estimate her or his level of activity.

The system encompasses the application running on different user end devices, for example, PDA, mobile phone, or a home computer. The application can perform number of tasks, given that it has established connection between the host and nodes, as well as interface to the user, and to the local server. The network architecture consists of network configuration and management system. The network configuration performs the following task: sensor node registration i.e. number of total nodes and their types, handshaking before initialization i.e. determining sample frequency and mode of operation, customization i.e. maintaining user specific and signal processing method, and secure the wireless communication i.e. encrypting and decrypting data. After the completing of WSN configuration, the applications take care of the network, manage the channel capacity of sharing, synchronizing clocks, data processing and transmitting, and storing the data in local server. Based on the network architecture of the network different medical nodes the application layer should determine the condition of the patient/ user and provide suggestions though an understandable graphical user interface. Lastly, if the nodes are available and secure to establish a connection, the information can be sent to medical server as a record or for later use.

The architecture includes medical sever connected via internet. In addition to the medical server, the last phase also consists of few other servers which provides commercial health care, telemedicine, remote monitoring, tracking server, and emergency server. The purpose of the medical sever is basically runs a server that sets up a communication between the channel and applications, store and collect the reports from the user end, and securely place the data into the medical server. Other servers can also offer E-health advice services to the user. This includes prescribing medicines or providing feedback to the patient correlating the information received. Depending on the stored data from the previous medical records of the user, all the services offer advice comparing the previous trends with the current trend of sensor data. The emergency server plays the role of notifying the doctors and the medical person in accordance with the level of emergency. Based on the level of emergency the response team takes immediate action. The hospital module monitors the patients remotely from the location of the patient, if the monitored patient is at home or a remote location. This module also allows analysis of all patients under monitoring centrally in the hospital or health care center.

2.1.3 System Design and Evaluation

Most of these wearable devices have maintained a standard before releasing: (1) Cost effective, (2) miniaturization of the module, and (3) low power consumption. With the development of IEEE 802.15.4/ZigBee and Bluetooth, tethered systems have become obsolete. The recent development of Bluetooth Low energy (BLE) creates an opportunity for making the system low power, low cost with high data rate applications. For home based remote monitoring, sensor data can be used with personal computer works as a data hub, and then it can store data via internet.

Recent advances in medical devices have lessened the frequency of physical checkup between patient and doctors. Since the user can upload the collected information directly to the cloud server, and doctors can easily monitor their patients in real time. However, existing systems are facing some major obstacle to make it more robust and user friendly. Current ECG electrodes use patches or adhesives to monitor patient, which creates discomfort if worn for a long period of time. It does not allow user to move and perform daily activities in a natural manner. Also gel electrodes are non-reusable, create irritation and can be the cause of skin allergies. In our proposed system we have used non-contact ECG electrodes from Plessy's Semiconductor Company. It works with both non-contact and contact manner. It is occupied with built in pre-amplifier. One drawback of capacitive-based electrodes is signals are not as strong as gel-based electrodes due to the high impedance of human skin and the fact that our bodies work as an antenna which affects noise in the signal. The significant factor of a capacitive-coupled ECG system is that even with a little displacement between the electrode and skin, and there will be a change in the coupling capacitance; hence, the signal will be distorted by motion.

Due to the bulkiness of the health monitoring devices most of the users are not comfortable to carry it on a daily basis. Although, with the help of highly integrated ICs and technical advancement, the size and weight of the devices has been shrunk dramatically. But patients, especially senior citizens are reluctant to use any kind additional devices for health monitoring. This can be achieved by integrating sensors with general purpose accessories like spectacles. Power consumption can be identified as one of the most pressing challenges of designing wearable's. As the wearable's are constrained by spaces, batteries must be as small as possible, hence power consumption of every component is critical. Using of BLE module and the power saving algorithm can save a significant amount of power. Not to mention, all the parameters have to be accurate and secure. Since the patient wants to secure the collected data to remain private, everything has to be encrypted and stored in a safe place. In terms of reliability medical devices have to be more reliable than any other general purpose systems. A small bug or failure in medical devices can be life threatening.

Compound of Wearable Technology: The wearable sensor network consists of three major components: (1) the sensor, which collects the physiological data and communicate with hardware, (2) the wireless network protocol to communicate between hardware and software, and (3) the processing unit to extract and analyze the data to a meaning level. Advancement in microelectronics, sensor development and data analysis technique has enabled the development of miniaturize wearable sensor for remote monitoring. Researchers have resolved above mentioned shortcomings in remote monitoring and improved the ambulatory technology that had previously established for scrutinizing patient's status. In Table 2.1 we have mentioned several types of sensor and their working method.

Minimizing the size of the sensor and electronics board of the sensor module has played a vital role in the development and deployment of the wearable systems. One of the major problems for the wearable sensor has been the size of the components and the development boards, recent advancement in power sources has also improved the life cycle of the modules. Previously it was very difficult to monitor patient for long span of time without having a bulky wearable system, but researchers have overcome this obstacle with integration of analog front end, sensors and microelectronics. A conceptual flexible circuit shown in Fig. 2.1 is an example of a wearable sensor node and allows to store and measure physiological data as well as transmit the data wirelessly with low power consumption. Sensors are used to analyze the health of the patient by measuring various bodily parameters. The sensors in the environment as well as on the patient should be small in size and as unobtrusive to the patient as possible for acquiring natural values of the parameters. The sensors include heart rate monitor, oximeter, blood pressure sensor, ECG module, and thermometer. These sensors produce raw values of data

Table 2.1 Different types of sensors and their working method

Sensors		
Physical	Chemical	Biological
1. Displacement	1. Composites	1. Antibody
2. Mass	2. Concentration	2. DNA
3. Force		3. Virus
4. Pressure		

Fig. 2.1 Conceptual wireless sensor node based on flexible circuit

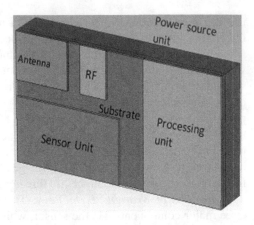

which are wirelessly relayed to a central transceiver unit worn by the patient. This transceiver unit processes the raw data and converts it into meaningful metadata (Md Shaad, 2015). Raw sensor data contains only values of the parameters measured hence has little value. Sensor Metadata when added to these values, viz. Type of parameter being monitored, feature of interest, timestamp and unit of measurement makes these values meaningful.

Physical: Physical sensors are used for measuring any kind of displacement, mass, force or pressure. The basic working principle is if there is any physical deformation of transducer, it exhibits changes as form of electrical charges. These information can be digitized using analog to digital converter and with right filtration method desired information can be stored. In recent years, different experiment has been done for these kind of sensors.

Chemical: These sensors can be used to identify the amplitude of giving concentration. Such as, presence of a particular gas in the air. When a gaseous molecule absorbs or added to graphite or carbon particle it changes its electrical properties, actually the number of electrons of the molecule gets increased or decreased. The output of the chemical change can also be converted into digital formation to quantify.

Biological: Biological sensors are used in observing the biological process like antibody, DNA, virus etc. These sensors are based on a biological recognition system and transduction mechanism. There are actually two types of biological sensor in terms of their working principle, one is electrochemical sensor and another is photometric sensors. Working principle of electrochemical sensor is similar to chemical sensor except the electrical changes is ignited by a protein or a specific antigen/antibody or a DNA that attach itself to metamaterials. It is able to detect virus, infections, asthma attacks, lung cancer or a parasitic element in the body. Another type of biological sensor is based on optical waves. When an optical wave's incident on a biological sensor it changes its resonance depends on the wavelength of the incident wave.

Power source is also a major concern for a wearable sensor node. In Hall (2009). They have constructed lithium Nano batteries, which has high power density with the dimension 200 nm. However, it needs to be recharged once in 10 days period, which is not feasible in case of nano-batteries. To eliminate this challenge energy harvesting has been introduced in the different research work. Energy harvesting can be achieved by-

Mechanical: When a surface moves or shake it can be converted into electrical energy. Energy can be harvested with muscle contraction or even with a heartbeat.

Vibration: It can be generated by EM waves or acoustic waves which can be used for harvesting energy.

Hydraulic: It is produced by oxygen or blood flow. To convert from one state of energy to another, zinc oxide nanowires based piezoelectric transducer can be used. When this transducer detects any kind of mechanical deformation there will be voltage changes in the nanowires. Moreover, this transducer can also detect vibration at a particular frequency. Therefore, this energy can be the power source of the system and can last for a life time or a really long period of time.

Cell phone technology plays a vital role when it comes to deigning wearable sensors, as it can be readily used as a hub for the network. Monitoring health with mobile phone as a central hub has been a commonplace for the wearable sensor designer. One of the major reason is its ubiquitous and easy to access. The global mobile phone has increased by 35 %, only in 2010 220 million phone has been shipped. Most of the smart phones are Android and IOS platform which is user friendly and developing an application is quite easy to communicate wirelessly with nodes. Moreover, it also can be used as processing the data and storing them in a secure place or the cloud. The pocket size mobile has more than enough processing power to compute all the complex algorithm for health monitoring and intervention applications.

The Central Transceiver Unit is a wearable module and can be attached to the patient. This is designed to receive the raw data from the wearable medical sensors through multiple channels tuned to multiple frequencies. Serialized transmission of data through one channel may cause delays or collisions, thus loss in data. Hence multiple channels are used to ensure that different sensors send their values at different frequencies separated by an offset value to prevent interference. This transceiver unit then transfers the processed metadata values to a central base station in the room using wireless communication like Zigbee or Bluetooth. The central base station gathers the values from the environmental sensors as well and then relays the data to the layer 2 as mentioned in the architecture in Section II. Hence, the Central Base Station acts as a gateway for the system between layer 1 and layer 2 of the architecture. The use of the central base station can be made cost effective and mobile if a smart device is used as the gateway being carried at all times by the patient. As we can see from the above discussion, during the last decade, we have witnessed the huge number of development of low power and miniaturized wearable devices. Most of these devices has maintained a standard before releasing: (1) Cost effective, (2) miniaturization of the module, and (3) low power consumption. With the development of IEEE 802.15.4/ZigBee and

Bluetooth, tethered systems have become obsolete. The recent development of Bluetooth Low energy (BLE) and IEEE 802.15.4a standard based on Ultra-wide-band (UWB) impulse radio creates an opportunity for making the system low power, low cost with high data rate applications. For home based remote monitoring, sensor data can be used with personal computer works as a data hub, and then it can store data via internet. A variety of mobile and ubiquitous healthcare solutions that were proposed for real time monitoring of ECG (Wang et al., 2010) (Fang, 2012) have been presented using technologies such as IEEE802.15.4 and the classical Bluetooth. Among those developed solutions IEEE802.15.4 served better the purpose by virtue of its attractive security and low energy consumption features when compared to classical Bluetooth. However the Bluetooth Special Interest group (SIG) has recently announced a new standard for low power personal area network devices named Bluetooth Low Energy (BLE) also referred as Bluetooth version 4. 0. Bluetooth 4.0 wireless technology is developed to provide features such as low-power, low latency, short-range and small-coin battery cell operation. It provides a maximum data rate of around 1 Mbps and supports a range of about 100 m, triggering its use for a wide range of applications with small form factors in industries such as healthcare, fitness, security and home entertainment. From above facts, it seems obvious that BLE offers more fascinating features when compared to IEEE802.15.4. However, its performance for such applications still needs to be determined.

2.2 Deployment Scenarios

The Wireless Body Area Networks (WBAN) can be deployed at home, in the workplace, or in hospitals. Wireless medical sensors attached to the user send data to a PDA, forming a short range wireless network (e.g., IEEE 802.15.1 or 802.15.3/4). The PDA equipped with a WLAN interface (e.g., IEEE 802.11a/b/g) transmits the data to the home (central) server. The home server, already connected to the Internet, can establish a secure channel to the medical server and send periodic updates for the user's medical record. The modified configuration in the middle is optimized for home health care. The sensor network coordinator is attached to the home personal server that runs the PS application. The medical sensor nodes and the network coordinator form a wireless personal area network. By excluding the PDA, we can reduce system cost. However, this setting is likely to require more energy spent for communication due to an increased RF output power and lower Quality of Service (QoS), requiring frequent retransmissions.

There are few requirements to fulfil wearable health monitoring system, such as wearability, reliable communication, Interoperability and security. To acquire non-contact and unobtrusive continuous monitoring, wireless sensors must be light and small in size. The bulkiness of the sensors is predominantly varied by the size and power of the batteries. However, the size of the battery is directly proportional to the capacity. In near future, we can expect to shrink down the battery along with integrated circuits which will improve the wearability of the medical sensor nodes. It is important to have a reliable wireless communication for WSN. The communication capacity varies with number with nodes and their sampling rate, varies from 1 to 1000 Hz. To improve the reliability, on-sensor processing can be done to reduce the time to process and transmit the data. Another important issue is overall system security. The problem of security arises at all layers of WSN for healthcare system. At the lowest level, wireless medical sensors must meet privacy requirements mandated by the law for all medical devices and must guarantee data integrity. Wireless medical sensors should allow users to easily assemble a robust WSN depending on the user's state of health.

2.3 Practical Implementation and Operating Challenges

In this section of the book, we will discuss about a practical design and implementation of a wearable device which can monitor ECG, heart rate, temperature, and fall detection of a chronic heart disease patient. Proposed wearable glass is interfaced with the Android application, where all data's can be stored in Secure Digital (SD) card or in a secure local server. The proposed system has been tested and verified with a breadboard prototype and a small PCB has been designed to demonstrate the actual system.

Development of Smart Glass for multiparameter health monitoring has been discussed in the section. The capacitive based non-contact sensor has a great interest in monitoring ECG signals, overcoming the disadvantages of traditional gel based electrodes. The overall system realizes 2 lead non-contact sensors, including following functions: (1) heart rate monitoring with the sampling precision of 12 bit (2) fall detection (3) Motion status in 3-axis accelerometer (4) sensing temperature (5) USB interface with integrated charging circuit and (6) supports Bluetooth low energy. The purpose of designing the system is to be used for long term monitoring and storage, so low power design has been taken into account.

(a) *System Design:*

Since the device is highly relying on ECG and motion data which does not require complex computation, the single chip wireless microcontroller has been used. Due to size-constrain and power consumption, we used Simblee, an ultra-low power wireless microcontroller manufactured by RF digital Co. This chip has a USB 2.0 interface to upload the programs, 12-bit analog to digital converter (ADC), provides serial communication which can be used as SPI and UART. The functional block diagram of the proposed device is shown in Fig. 2.2.

The system also consists of 3.7 V Li-ion battery with rechargeable circuit. Three sensors have been used so far ECG electrodes, temperature and motion sensor. The analog front end (AFE) comprised with multiple stages of amplifier and filters. A 3-axis accelerometer has also been utilized for motion detection. And a built in Simblee temperature sensor has been used. These analog values are then

Fig. 2.2 A block diagram of
the wearable system

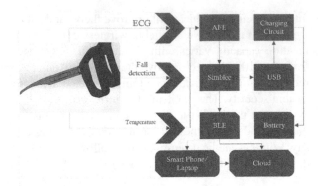

converted to a digital signal by ADC, then send it to host through Bluetooth 4.0. The ECG, temperature and motion information directly displayed on the smartphone screen in real-time. Based on the customer requirements more sensors can be added to this device for example infrared sensor for measuring SpO2. In addition, different algorithms can be implemented to track sleep pattern and efficiency of daily activities. The data transmission can also take in both wired and wireless methods. The proposed system is carefully designed so that it can be adapted to fulfill the customer requirement. For the designated target group of cardiac patients, the vital signs need to be monitored are ECG, respiration and heart rate. In addition, having the information about motion and temperature makes it more reliable. For ECG monitoring, the patient must be physically connected to the ECG electrodes. However, recent advancement of sensor development has enabled to make non-contact ECG sensors. Direct contact sensors have protection circuit and also need isolation to avoid high current flow, which makes it complex to design.

(b) *Custom Analog Front End (AFE):*

Special care for low power and high input impedance was taken in the AFE. Originally it was foreseen to combine AFE and wireless microprocessor with power unit with custom made printed circuit board. Unfortunately the due to manufacturing process the final prototype was not ready by the project end. However, with low power design, the power consumption is still below 17 mAh and it would be lower with the final version.

The purpose of the AFE is to extract, amplify, and filter small bio-potential signal in the presence of different noise sources. The active electrodes were placed two sides of the forehead to extract the ECG signal without any physical contact. For high input impedance, a buffer circuit is added to the front end, analog circuit and proper shielding was used to reduce the electromagnetic interference. The front end circuit consists of a pair of PS25255; which has built in amplifier. The front end circuit starts with a buffer amplifier LMP7701 which helps to improve the input impedance and bootstraps the biasing network. The output signal is connected to AD8221, an ultra-high input impedance instrumental amplifier. This provides the differential gain and drives the common line. The multiple HPF and LPF have been used to reduce the low and high frequency components. The analog circuit is designed for optimal performance with very low power consumption. A 60 Hz notch filter is also used to remove baseline fluctuation noises. The DRL circuit is connected to a virtual ground, which act as a reference voltage for all amplifiers and filters.

(c) *Simblee: Wireless Processing Unit*

Most of the people do not use BLE because it is relatively new, but it provides great range medical application. BLE can also be sued as a payment method as it is secure, localized and easy to use. BLE can sync and communicate with the other BLE host. In our case we have used Simblee RFD77101, it was released in late 2015 by RF Digital Co. It is a high performance, professional grade Bluetooth 4.0 transceiver with built in 32-bit ARM Cortex M0 processor. This processor can be programmed with Arduino IDE with Simblee package or with over the air (OTA). Simblee is also known as IoT4EE (IoT for Everyone and Everything). Unlike other IoT devices, Simblee can directly upload GUI description code to the cell phone. The operating voltage is 1.8–3.6 V and can communicate with other devices from a few centimeters to 50 m. It has 29 general purpose input/output (GPIO) and 10-bit analog to digital converter (ADC), which perfectly fits in our project. Simblee does not only make the developing path easy it also has very low latency and its timing accuracy is extremely promising. The size of it is so small and inexpensive which can easily utilize in embedded system. To connect the Simblee module to a computer, it uses Gazell or GZLL protocol, which was developed by Nordic Semiconductor. With this protocol device can only communicate with the host, so inter device communication cannot be achieved.

(d) *Software Algorithm:*

The firmware handles all the control and computation operations. The firmware was based on Arduino programming language and we have used IDE 1.6.5 to compile and upload the firmware. It also has a power saver mode; instead of transmitting data all the time it collects only when there is a request from the user. Although it has woken up delay but saves the power consumption. Another important aspect of this experiment is where the signals are originating from. Our head, is a good source for the ECG and EEG signal, hence proposed system is more stable and robust. To visualize the analog signal in the computer, a graphical user interface is used, which is developed in Processing software. For mobile phone interface, we have a custom build Android applications for Simblee. Although RF Digital has reference to IOS application, but until now there has been no Android application. We have developed an Android based application to talk to Simblee and perform all the desired computation. It also includes the software level manipulation too, but at a minor level, so that we can see the real time simulation. However, for PC based applications we implemented FFT to reduce the noise the signal, it also includes amplification and filtration. As Simblee works with only Bluetooth 4.0 laptop or PC cannot be connected with stock Bluetooth 2.0. So, with another Simblee connected to PC can talk to each other with GZLL protocol. We utilize built in ADC of Simblee to convert the analog signal and

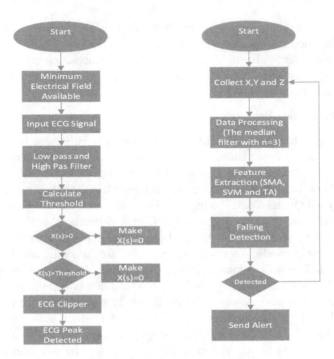

Fig. 2.3   Overall flow chart for ECG peak and fall detection

digital signal coming from AFE. When the device is powered on, main program receives the data for electrical field, means if there are voltage changes in analog pin, the program will start to work. Then it initializes AD converter, timer, SPI and Bluetooth. Figure 2.3 shows the flowchart of collecting ECG and fall detection. The ECG threshold is calculated based on the average of the incoming signal. There are many peak detection methods available to date. In our project, we utilized the most general method to make it easier and more energy efficient. With this method, it is easy to manipulate false positive and false negative signals. The R-R intervals can be calculated from peak to peak signals. Band pass was filtered at 40 Hz and Q = 0.707 was multiplied by all of the data for the desired interval. Furthermore, these data sets are multiplied by 3 to get beats per minute (BPM).

   Head and waist are relevant area for fall detection, using simple threshold and posture classification. Cellphone can recognize fall detection by the values of x, y and z form accelerometer, but the classification is much more complex and not easy to implement. Whereas head is the perfect position for fall detection with high accuracy. All body movements can categorize with below 20 Hz frequency, including movement due to body motion, gravitational acceleration, external vibration and environmental noise. Feature extraction can be done using Tilt Angle (TA), pastoral orientation refers to the body tilt angle to the normal. As the below equation states, it's the angle between positive y-axis and the gravitational vector g. The system will trigger an interrupt if the value of the TA is below 40°.

Fig. 2.4 3D prototype of the wearable glass and custom made PCB with non-contact ECG electrode (Md Shaad Mahmud, 2016)

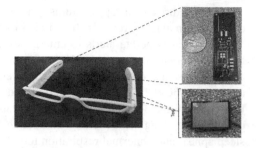

$$TA = \arcsin(\frac{Yi}{\sqrt{Xi^2 + Yi^2 + Zi^2}})$$

(e) *Prototyping:*

A 3D model is shown in Fig. 2.4, it was designed using the student version of Autodesk Inventor. The wearable glass was designed with measurements from PS252555 sensor and the PCB. The lithium ion battery we use for PCB is from all-battery website, with a size of $10 \times 5 \times 2$ mm. In case of heart failure or fall detection an SOS signal will be sent to the authorities along with SMS, voice signal and location. The first prototype was developed with the help of 3D printer in our facility. The material of the case was printed using ABS material.

We have developed an Android application to communicate with the sensors through Simblee. There are several aspects of the app. As this application aims to achieve successful communication with our system, it introduces a number of features. But before going to that we need to discuss how we achieved transmission between sensor and Simblee. In order to connect the app need to run on Android phones that have BLE capability which starts from Android 4.3 (API Level 18). Our application needs to connect to different profiles as we need various sensor data. So we scan the device based on different service UUID. Once we discover our intended device with service UUID we establish a Generic Attribute Profile (GATT) connection with the device. The next step is getting the characteristics of the service. One of the characteristics contains the descriptor that we need to set true in order to receive the data. The 128 bit UUIDs that we used in connecting the device are listed as:

UUID_SERVICE=0000fe84-0000-1000-8000-00805F9B34FB (for heart rate),

0000fe85-0000-1000-8000-00805F9B34FB (for temperature)

UUID_RECEIVE=2d30c082-f39f-4ce6-923f 3484ea480596 (characteristic UUID)

UUID_SEND = 2d30c083-f39f-4ce6-923f-3484ea480596

UUID_DISCONNECT =2d30c084-f39f-4ce6-923f-3484ea480596

UUID_CLIENT_CONFIGURATION=00002902-0000-1000-8000-00805f9b34fb

(descriptor UUID)

Now we discuss our app features. The mobile app receives heart rate from the device and maintains records. It can also look for unusual heart rates and if configured, it can generate alerts to emergency contacts with the location. ECG and heart rate monitoring can provide very important information's. Patients to record of cardiovascular diseases such as supraventricular tachycardia (SVT) or CHF (congestive heart failure) can be monitored and get help in cases of emergency. Detection of acute events like atrial fibrillation and MI (myocardial infarctions) can be done along with seeking immediate helps. It provides information about sleep apneas and abnormal respiration too. Activity monitoring is highly useful for providing a snapshot of the total daily activity. The device also reports fall to the cell phone in real time. With the signal specified for fall, it sends an immediate message to their emergency contact points. It is very useful for the elderly persons and those who requires assisted living. The app records the temperature data from the device. It can alert the user on temperature readings beyond this threshold (Fig. 2.5).

(f) *Results and Discussion:*

Several measurements were conducted with the developed prototype to demonstrate the ECG and heart rate signal with a non-contact and contact method. A 25 years old person's physiological data were taken in our department's laboratory to validate the results in real time.

Although a non-contact sensor is the most convenient sensor to measure ECG, when compared to wet contact electrodes. However, it is much complicated to measure and susceptible to motion art effects. Hence, the effectiveness of the ECG electrodes plays a vital role in case of non-contact measurement. Therefore, the effectiveness of the electrodes is crucial. Typically the generated signal is in the range of 1 mV. AFE for non-contact sensors has to be designed carefully so that

Fig. 2.5 Developed Android app, **a** front UI of developed application, **b** ECG signals coming from wearable glass

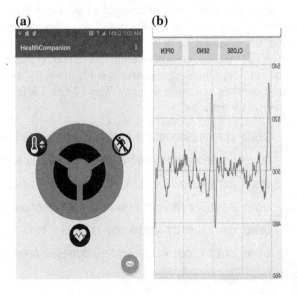

we get maximum capacitive deflection, so there are three major factors to keep in mind. Firstly, the large surface area of the electrodes; the bigger the surface area, the more capacitance you will get, hence strong signals. Secondly, reducing the gap between the electrode and skin; the less distance you have between skin and conductor, the better result you will get. Thirdly, the insulator of skin and the conductor has to have a high dielectric constant. The proposed system has been proven to be a robust and stable sensor node. Figure 2.6 shows the system setup of the front end, analog circuit with AFE, Simblee and an accelerometer.

The overall quality of the signal was good. As for our case, the separation between the sensor and skin was almost constant which creates a surprisingly good result. One of the disadvantages of non-contact sensor is susceptible to moving effect. Just moving the wiring could cause distortion in signals. There are still more testing and experiments has to be done to compete with medical grade devices.

Figure 2.7 shows the results of the proposed ECG system, Fig. 2.7a is the direct output from the PS25255 ECG sensor. The input impedance of this system is more than 10 Gohm. Figure 2.7b is the analog output from AFE. As the power consumption is very important for continuous monitoring, we calculated power consumption for each component of the system. AFE only takes about 3.7 % of the total power. To do this, voltage was supplied by a DC source and the current has been calculated from an oscilloscope. Power is then just a multiplication of the voltage and current for each part, which we compared from the total supply. Then Fig. 2.7c is the final output of the system calculated from a PC based software. The light gray line in the middle is the reference voltage to detect peaks. On top of the screen, it also shows the beats per minute (BPM). Output signals are quite easily detectable and shows competitive results compare to current fitness tracking devices like fitbit, Jawbone etc. However, one factor common to all these

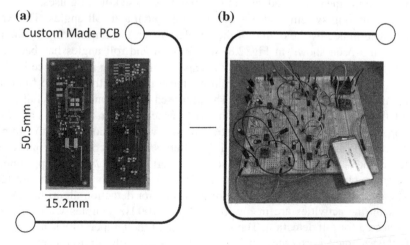

Fig. 2.6 Fully integrated miniaturized PCB, **a** top and bottom part of the custom made PCB, **b** 1st prototype of the hardware system

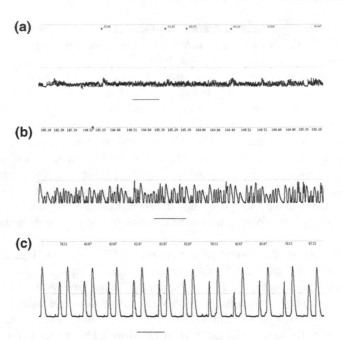

Fig. 2.7 Output signal ECG sensor from different source. **a** Raw analog signal directly coming from PS25255 sensor without any filtration, **b** output signal of AFE with 500 mV peak voltage, **c** Filtered output signal of the system electrodes placed on wearable glass with 1 V peak voltage

experiments is the motion art effects, which is inevitable in the case of a capacitance-based, non-contact sensor. Every time the subject moves, the capacitance will change with it, resulting in noise with the original signal. In future research, we will be implementing an adaptive filter to reduce these kind of noises.

The monitoring system analyzes acceleration, pitch and roll angles. The RMS value is determined by the output of the accelerometer. Data measuring by the fall detection has been shown in Fig. 2.8, where pitch and roll angles has been displayed. The motion of the human body is capable of bringing interference in ECG signal. Our research is going on to remove these noises with adaptive filter and display the filtered ECG in real-time. The proposed system can monitor fall detection of the patient, it is equipped with 3-axis accelerometer. LIS3DH chip from ST Corporation is selected as the motion sensor, which is connected to Simblee through the SPI interface. The free fall detection is internal configured in accelerometer, in the case of fall detection it sends an alert signal to Android app running on the smart phone. For fall detection the accelerometer coordinates do not have to fix, only magnitude of the sum vector is needed for detection algorithm. As for the human, the activities are in low frequencies, 100 Hz samples with ± 2 g has been selected for fall detection. The sole purpose of the temperature sensor was to verify the accuracy. Fortunately, it has been successful with minimum error.

Fig. 2.8 Pitch and Roll angles during a forward fall ending up lying with recovery

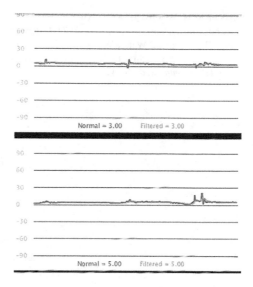

The proposed method includes non-contact sensor with low power consumption based on Simblee and a fully integrated AFE, which can monitor patients ECG, heart rate and respiration continuously. Also, this system is equipped with an acceleration sensor and supports Bluetooth 4.0 communication, and could monitor patient motion, physical activity and fall detection. There has been some research carried out using non-contact sensors, but most of them suffered due to a motion effect, and hence are not suitable for medical grade applications. In this paper, we carefully designed non-contact ECG sensors, which is comparable to standard Ag/AgCl electrodes. However, the acceleration sensor can be used to implement the adaptive filter which can minimize noise from motion art effects. As the working frequency of medical devices is in the range of 0.01–3 Hz (maximum), it gets very easy noise and interference; therefore, filtering, amplifying and separating analog signals needs to be taken carefully dealt with. There are also some problems regarding materials, packaging, miniaturization, signal processing and prediction theory which need to be addressed and adequately solved. Future research will encompass a system eliminating all of these issues.

References

Fang, Z. Z. (2012). ECG-cryptography and authentication in body area networks. *IEEE Transactions on Information Technology in Biomedicine*, 1070–1078.

Hall, M. M. (2009). Nano structure carbons for energy storage in lithium oxygen batteries. In *2009 International Conference on Sustainable Power Generation and Supply*. IEEE.

Md Shaad Mahmud, H. E. (2016). A real time and non-contact multiparameter wearable device for health monitoring. In *IEEE Global Communications (GLobecom)*. DC: IEEE.

Md Shaad, H. W. (2015). An inexpensive and ultra-low power sensor node for wireless health monitoring system. In *IEEE HealthCOM*. IEEE.

Wang, H., Peng, D., Wang, W., Sharif, H., Chen, H. H., & Khoynezhad, A. (February 2010). Resource-aware secure ECG healthcare monitoring through body sensor networks. *IEEE Wireless Communication*, 12–19.

Chapter 3
Architecture

3.1 Remote Healthcare Monitoring Architecture

3.1.1 Sensor Network Architecture

Sensors are basic components for all sensor networks, and their quality depends heavily on industry advances in signal conditioning and processing, microelectromechanical systems (MEMS), and nanotechnology. Sensors are classified into three categories: physiological, biokinetic, ambient environmental sensors.

Physiological sensors measure physiological vital signs such as blood pressure, heart rate, glucose level, core body temperature, blood oxygen, and respiratory rate. Physiological vital signs are the measures of various physiological statistics acquired by WBSN in order to assess the most basic body functions of patients. The vital signs taking normally involves recording body temperature, heart rate, blood pressure, and respiratory rate, but it may also include other measurements such as posture and motion, pulse oximetry and electrocardiography (ECG). For biomedical measurements such as pressure, flow and temperature, and various sensors can be adopted to meet the common medical measurand characteristics, which are listed in Table 3.1.

Only a few medical signals such as body temperature are constant or varying very slowly. These biosensors are converting biosignals that are function of time, that is biosignals are dynamic not static in nature. Thus, biomeasurement systems together with sensors should be considered from the stand point of dynamic instrument characteristics. Instruments are described by a linear differential equation relating output signal to input signal in time domain.

© The Author(s) 2016
H. Wang et al., *Wireless Health*, SpringerBriefs in Computer Science,
DOI 10.1007/978-3-319-47946-0_3

Table 3.1 Biomedical measured characteristics

Measurement	Range of parameter	Frequency, Hz	Sensor or method
Blood flow	1–300 mL/s	0–20	Flow meter
Blood pressure	0–400 mmHg	0–50	Strain gauge or cuff
Electrocardiography	0.5–5 mV	0.05–150	Skin electrodes
Electroencephalography	5–300 μV	0.5–150	Scalp electrodes
Electromyography	0.1–5 mV	0–10000	Needle electrode
pH	3–13	0–1	pH electrode
Respiratory rate	2–50 breaths/min	0–10	Impedance, fiber optic
Temperature	32–40 °C	0–0.1	Thermistor, thermocouple

3.1.2 Big Data Infrastructure and Cloud Computing (Fang et al., 2015)

Big data are defined in various ways, but the three "V" features are their common characteristics: volume (large datasets), variety (different types of data from myriad sources), and velocity (data collected in real time). Variability and complexity are considered as two other features, especially by those focusing on analytics. Big data require new forms of processing to enable enhanced decision making, insight discovery, and process optimization. These large-scale data can be produced on the web, by sensors, or by monitoring systems (Bollier & Firestone, 2010). For example, 2.7 zetabytes of data exist in the digital universe; 235 terabytes of data were collected by the U.S. Library of Congress in April 2011; business transactions on the Internet, business-to-business and business-to-consumer, will reach 450 billion per day by the year 2020. The term big data is also used to capture the opportunities and challenges facing all researchers in accessing, managing, analyzing, and integrating datasets of diverse data types. The rapid growth in data size and scope created a need for multi-disciplinary collaboration and joint efforts from industries, academics, and governments to develop novel methods, disciplines, and workforces that can blend data networking, management, computational, and statistical sciences. This multi-disciplinary collaboration initiative was launched at the prestigious 2014 Joint Statistical Meetings, American Statistical Association, where top computer scientists, engineers, and statisticians share their respective approaches to Big Data models, algorithms, and networks (H. Fang et al.).

Web-based and mobile health intervention studies have the advantages of combining tailored approaches of face-to-face interventions with the scalability of public health interventions via the Internet with lower cost (htt). It is a promising solution for healthcare due to its accessibility and time and cost savings. They have been developed for the following clinical areas:

- Chronic conditions, such as heart disease, arthritis, and asthma.
- Health promotion, such as alcohol reduction, smoking cessation, diet, and exercise.
- Mental health, such as anxiety and depression.

For example, MAPIT, a web-based intervention system targeting substance abuse treatment in the criminal justice system, has been developed. It includes the extended parallel process model, motivational interviewing, and social cognitive theory. A web-based personally controlled health management system, Health.me, integrates an untethered personal health record with consumer care pathways and social forums to support healthcare. Caring Web has been introduced to support family caregivers of persons with stroke residing in home settings. An innovative web-based system has been developed to allow patient-reported outcome measures to be easily administered. It can also be used for any medical intervention. The performance of a web-based intervention for mild to moderate depression, namely MoodGYM program, is evaluated. The usability of Tobacco Tractics, a website for reducing tobacco usage, is studied. However, the analytics for unstructured big data from these web-based and mobile health interventions are underdeveloped, because they are usually spatially-varied and temporally-varied data with missing values. Trajectory pattern recognition approaches are being initiated, developed and verified for such studies at the University of Massachusetts Medical School, such as the DISC project funded by the National Institute of Health (NIH) (htt1).

Big data has the potential to improve behavioral medicine research and outcomes. Big Data to Knowledge (BD2K) is an initiative that aims to develop new approaches, standards, methods, tools, software, and competencies that will enhance the use of biomedical big data. The national library of Medicine is also promoting the use of common data elements to support sharing of big data. Integrative data analysis (the pooling of independent data sets that can be analyzed as one) was promoted as one of the techniques in behavioral medicine. At the 2014 annual meeting of the Society of Behavioral Medicine, pattern recognition for big data was emphasized. The aforementioned DISC project proposed the trajectory pattern recognition approach to behavioral interventions.

Linking big administrative data sets, such as the National Death Index, Medicare and Medicaid enrollment claims, and Social Security Administration Retirement and Disability data, to national health surveys (e.g. National Health Interview Survey (NHIS), National Health and Nutrition Examination Survey (NHANES), The Second Longitudinal Study of Aging (LSOA II), National Nursing Home Survey (NNHA)) is also challenging. The linkage methodologies are called on to examine issues such as health status, health conditions, healthcare, and health behaviors.

Big data includes unstructured data coming from sensors, devices, third parties, web applications, and social media, in real time and on a large scale. SAS provides four kinds of big data solutions: data management, high performance analytics, high performance data visualization, and flexible deployment options. A comprehensive data management approach is offered in these solutions to allow any amount of data to be managed, analyzed, and visualized effectively. EMC insists that vision, talent, and technology are required to make big data a success, providing solutions to big data management and analysis. GigaSpaces builds and deploys a large-scale real-time analytics system using big data technologies where customers are able to handle scalability, performance and database integration seamlessly by providing simple event processing business logic.

IBM is using big data technologies to harness individual data resources in healthcare. Their approaches include building sustainable healthcare systems, collaborating to improve care and outcomes, and increasing access to healthcare. Infosys Labs is building the following:

1. Big Data Medical Engine in the Cloud (BDMEiC), a new Health Doctor that uses the method of diagnosing, customizing, and administering health care in real time using BDMEiC.
2. Big Data Powered Extreme Content Hub, which uses the approach of taming the big content explosion and providing contextual and relevant information.
3. Nature Inspired Visualization of Unstructured Big Data, which reconstructs self-organizing maps as spider graphs for better visual interpretation of large unstructured datasets. GNS is discovering healthcare methods through big data.

Its analytics solutions are being applied across the healthcare industry from pharmaceutical and biotechnology companies to integrated delivery systems and accountable care organizations (ACOs).

3.1.3 Data Analytics for Biomedical Big Data (Zhang & Fang, 2016)

Web-delivered trials are an important component in eHealth services. These trials, mostly behavior-based, generate big heterogeneous data that are longitudinal, high dimensional with missing values. Unsupervised learning methods have been widely applied in this area, however, validating the optimal number of clusters has been challenging. Built upon our multiple imputation (MI) based fuzzy clustering, MIfuzzy, we proposed a new multiple imputation based validation (MIV) framework and corresponding MIV algorithms for clustering big longitudinal eHealth data with missing values, more generally for fuzzy-logic based clustering methods. Specifically, we detect the optimal number of clusters by auto-searching and synthesizing a suite of MI-based validation methods and indices, including conventional (bootstrap or cross-validation based) and emerging (modularity-based) validation indices for general clustering methods as well as the specific one (Xie and Beni) for fuzzy clustering. The MIV performance was demonstrated on a big longitudinal dataset from a real web-delivered trial and using simulation. The results indicate MI-based Xie and Beni index for fuzzy-clustering is more appropriate for detecting the optimal number of clusters for such complex data. The MIV concept and algorithms could be easily adapted to different types of clustering that could process big incomplete longitudinal trial data in eHealth services.

In eHealth services, web-delivered trials or interventions are in increasing demand due to their cost-effective potential in accessing a large population (Eysenbach, 2011). These trials commonly generate big, complex, heterogenous and high-dimensional longitudinal data with missing values. These data have the typical five "V" properties of big data (Fang et al., 2015). Specifically, the Volume of such data is substantially large in terms of the number of participants and attributes, with which traditional clinical trials are incomparable; its Variety refers to different web-delivered components; its Velocity is undoubtly superior to traditional offline trials, because the data are recorded real-time; its Veracity is obvious because of its unstructured nature and messiness; and its Value would be substantial as long as its efficacy is clarified.

Our line of research focuses on multiple imputation based fuzzy clustering (MIfuzzy), as it fits better to longitudinal behavioral trial data than other methods based on our previous studies (Fang et al., 2009). There is a paucity of literature in validating the clustering results from big longitudinal eHealth trial data with missing values and our line of research (Zhang, Fang, & Wang, 2015) attempts to fill this gap. Probabilistic clustering (e.g., Gaussian Mixture models) and Hidden Markov Model-based Bayesian clustering, Neural networks models (e.g., Kohonen's Self Organizing Map, SOM), Hierarchical clustering, Partition-based clustering (e.g., K-means or Fuzzy C Means) are commonly used for clustering and demonstrated efficiently for specific data structure in other fields. However, these methods have at least one of these following disadvantages and are less appealing to big behavioral trial data which are typically high dimensional, heterogeneous, non-normal, longitudinal with missing values: Assumption of underlying statistical distributions (Gaussian) or prior distributions (Bayesian approach); (slow) convergence to a local maximum or no convergence at all especially for multi-modal distributions and large proportions of missing values with high-dimensional data and many clusters; unclear validation indices or procedures; inability to handle missing values or incorporate information about the shape and size of clusters; computational inefficiency; and their unknown utility in behavioral trial studies. With a pre-specified number of clusters, MI-Fuzzy was demonstrated to perform better than these methods in terms of its clustering accuracy and inconsistency rates using real trial data.

As aforementioned, missing data are common in longitudinal trial studies (Little & Rubin, 2014) (Schafer, 1997). The performance of MI-Fuzzy was evaluated under these three mechanisms: Missing Completely at Random, Missing at Random (MAR) and Missing not at Random (NMAR). The preliminary results indicate that MIfuzzy is invariant to the three mechanisms and accounts for the clustering uncertainty in comparison to non- or single-imputed fuzzy clustering (Zhang & Fang, 2016).

Built upon our multiple imputation (MI) based fuzzy clustering, MIfuzzy, we proposed MI-based validation framework (MIV) and corresponding MIV algorithms for clustering such big longitudinal web-delivered trial data with missing values. Briefly, MIfuzzy is a new trajectory pattern recognition method with a full integration and enhancement of multiple imputation theory for missing data and fuzzy logic theories. Here, we focus on cluster validation and extend traditional validation of complete data to MI-based validation of incomplete big longitudinal data, especially for fuzzy-logic based clustering (Acock, 2005). Unlike simple imputation such as mean, regression, and hot deck that cause bias and lose statistical precision, multiple-imputation accounts for imputation uncertainty (Buck, 1960).

To build the MIV, we consider two clustering stability testing methods, cross-validation and bootstrapping; to adapt to fuzzy clustering, we use Xie and Beni (XB), a widely-accepted fuzzy clustering validation index, and another newly emerging index, modularity.

Clustering stability has been used in recent years to help select the number of clusters. It measures the robustness against the randomness of clustering results. The core idea is based on the intuition that a good clustering will produce a stable result that does not vary from one sample to another. The clustering stability method can be used in both distance based and non-distance based clustering methods, such as model based clustering and spectrum clustering. Bootstrap and cross-validation are two common clustering stability testing methods. Bootstrap is a statistical technique to assign measures of accuracy, such as bias, variance and confidence intervals, to sample estimates. Bootstrap is used when the sampling size is small or impossible to draw repeated samples from the population of interest. In such cases, bootstrap can be used to approximate the sampling distribution of a statistic (Bickel, 1981). Cross-validation can be used in clustering algorithms to estimate its predictive strength (Shao, 1993). In cross-validation, the data is split to two or more partitions. Some partitions are used for training the model parameters, and the others, namely the validation (testing) set, are used to measure the performance of the model.

Two types of cross-validation can be distinguished, exhaustive and non-exhaustive: The first one includes leave-p-out and leave-one-out cross-valuation; the latter does not compute all ways of splitting the original data. The non-exhaustive cross-validation contains k-fold cross-validation, holdout and repeated random sub-sampling validation. The holdout method is the simplest among cross-validation methods, with which the data set is only separated into one training and one testing set. Although computationally efficient, the evaluation may be significantly different depending on how the division of the dataset is made between the training and testing sets. The k-fold cross validation improves and generalizes the holdout method by dividing a dataset into k subsets, where the variance of the resulting estimate is reduced as k is increased. A variant of this method is called repeated random sub-sampling validation, also known as Monte Carlo cross-validation to randomly divide the data into a test and training set k different times. Due to randomness, some data may never be selected while others may be selected more than once, resulting in potential overlapped validation subsets. The k-fold cross validation was used in this work to ensure that all data points are used for both training and validation, and each data point is used for validation exactly once. Modularity can measure the structure of networks or graphs, and can be used to cluster data by transforming the data points into a graph with their similarities. Thus, modularity can be used to determine the number of clusters in data analyses.

Most importantly, for fuzzy clustering, Xie and Beni (Xie & Beni, 1991), this widely accepted validation fuzzy clustering index was incorporated into this MI validation framework.

We proposed MIV algorithms to auto-search, compare, synthesize and detect the optimal number of clusters for incomplete big longitudinal data based on MI-based clustering stability tests (MI-cross-validation and MI-bootstrapping), MI-XB, and MI-modularity. The rest of the paper is organized as follows: Section "Multiple-imputation"—In eHealth services, big data from web-delivered longitudinal trials are complex. Determining the optimal number of clusters in such data is especially challenging. This paper built upon our MIfuzzy clustering designed a MI-based validation (MIV) framework and algorithms for big data processing, particularly for fuzzy clustering of big incomplete longitudinal web-delieved trial data. Although we included two conventional methods for testing clustering stability, bootstrap and cross-validation, they did not seem to add incremental value for detecting the optimal number of clusters. One major reason could be that the multiple imputation component in MIfuzzy already accounts for the imputation uncertainty to ensure the clustering stability using several complete imputed datasets. This concept is similar to the bootstrap and cross validation for stability tests, therefore this overlap decreases the incremental value of these conventional methods which are typically used for complete data sets. Another reason might be that the two methods were not specifically designed for or directly related to the fuzzy clustering which is widely accepted for biomedical data where clusters overlap or touch. Also the modularity validation index is widely accepted for network-based data, but appears not feasible for the structure of these big incomplete longitudinal web-delivered trial data in eHealth services. Consistently, we found multiple-imputation based XB index, specifically designed for fuzzy clustering, could facilitate detecting the optimal number of clusters for big incomplete longitudinal trial data, either from web-delivered or traditional clinical trials. Different from the MI approach used for statistical analyses, MI based clustering only uses the imputation step, thus has no connection with the possible inconsistent analytical models for statistical inference. As our research indicates, it will especially contribute more to non-model-based clustering approaches, and could potentially improve clustering accuracy and computational efficiency for model-based clustering approaches. In future, embedding MIV algorithms into eHealth system could warrant the validity of identifying at-risk or abnormal patterns of patients, events, diagnoses or services using various unsupervised learning methods, and reduce the uncertainty in implementing pattern-derived adaptive trials or services.

3.2 Secure and Smart and Connected Health

3.2.1 Connected Health Architecture

In recent years, the development of WBANs technology has been driven by pressure to reduce the health care cost, and support disease prevention and early risk

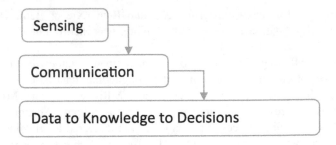

Fig. 3.1 Connected health structure

detection. WBANs can be deployed on a person's body for pervasive and real-time healthcare monitoring in the form of multimedia such as text, audio, image and video. The non-intrusive and ambulatory health monitoring of patients' vital signs over WBANs provides an economical solution to the current healthcare system, in which the health-care information can be distributed to users anytime through handheld devices and internet. A WBANs consists of a set of mobile and small size intercommunicating sensors, which are either wearable or can be implanted into the human body for monitoring vital signs (e.g., heart rate, brain activity, blood pressure and oxygen saturation) and/or environmental parameters (e.g., location, temperature, humidity and light) and movements (Fig. 3.1).

However, there are several challenges before WBANs can be widely deployed. First, the security and privacy issues: the data transmission in WBANs should be secure and accurate. The patient data is only derived from each patient's dedicated WBAN and is not mixed up with other patient's data. Further, The data from WBANs should have secure and limited access. The lack of security in the operation and communication of resource-constrained medical sensor nodes in WBANs have been an obstacle to move the technology forward. Second, the interference issue: the WBANs should function well even in dense deployment scenario, such as in a school or hospital. They will interference with each other due to limited available frequency bands. The interference decline the signal to interference plus noise Ratio (SINR) and thereby cause throughput degradation and more packet loss, which leads to energy waste. It should be noted that energy is the scarcest resource in WBAN due to most sensors in WBANs use battery, which has limited power supply. The challenges with the use of WBANs also includes interoperability, battery technology, sensor technology, and data management.

A typical topology of WBANs includes multiple types of medical sensors that can be wirelessly connected to other medical sensors or to the control nodes (e.g., Smart-phones), which could interface with other types of networks such as WiMAX or WiFi to further deliver the collected medical information to the information center. Many great efforts have been devoted to developing secure communication schemes between the internet and control nodes. Thus, our studies focus on the securing inter-sensor communication over the body area instead. A comprehensive survey on wireless body area networks is given in (Chen, Gonzalez, Vasilakos, Cao, & Leung, 2011).

Besides the transitional key distribution schemes, there are several on-going research works that implement the key distribution using biometric features. The research in (Venkatasubramanian, Banerjee, & Gupta, 2008) utilize the physiological signals for securing intersensor communication over WBANs. The authors in (Venkatasubramanian et al., 2008) proposed the use of the frequency coefficients of the ECG or Photoplethysmogram (PPG) signals to generate cryptographic keys. In (Bao, Zhang, & Shen, 2005), the Inter-Pulse-Interval (IPI) derived from ECG/PPG signals is proposed to generate cryptographic keys.

One solution to support secure communication is using prior key distribution. However, this method need human intervention and it is inconvenient when adding new sensors or replacing current ones. Using biometric information to secure the wireless communication is promising in WBAN applications. It does not need prior key distribution and use dynamic keys. Paper (Venkatasubramanian, Banerjee, & Gupta, 2010) (H. Wang) proposed to use ECG/EKG as a seed to generate a random key which is used to secure the wireless channel. The method in (Zhang, Wang, Vasilakos, & Fang, 2012) also need extra hardware though it uses an Improved Juels and Sudan algorithm to avoid the communication overhead brought in by Fuzzy Vault algorithm.

The PSKA scheme uses Fuzzy Vault to lock the randomly generated key in the vault at the sender, and unlock the vault to regenerate the key by the similar features available at the receiver. However, the security of the vault depend on its size, so extra Chaff points are needed to ensure the security of the vault, which brings the extra communication overheads. The authors of paper (Biel, Pettersson, Philipson, & Wide, 2001) suggest the use of ECG signals as a biometric feature to authenticate users and messages. The approach requires the creation of an ECG template and then comparing their current ECG signals with this template to verify the identity. However, it is not efficient to achieve good security performance due to using the static template. Besides using the biometric for securing the wireless channel, in recent years, researchers are studying the feasibility of using the wireless channel information to secure the communication.

In our work, we proposed an ECG-IJS authentication and encryption algorithm, by which the time-variant features are extracted from the ECG signals and used as keys to encrypt/authenticate messages. In the ECG-IJS scheme, both the sender and receiver node need to be coupled with an additional ECG sensors. This requirement causes hardware cost and extra-energy consumption. To address this problem, we also proposed CIAE, a channel information based cryptography and authentication scheme, for WBANs applications. The proposed CIAE uses dynamic keys and works in a ply-n-play manner. We also proposed a feature generation methods which needs a longer channel sampling when channel changes slowly to provide key variations.

We studied the authentication and encryption problem for WBANs. We first proposed ECG-IJS, an ECG-based authentication and encryption algorithm to secure the wireless data transmission for WBANs. Features are generated from ECG signals and further used as keys to encrypted the transmitting data at sender. The sender send the encrypted data and "helper" information to the receiver. After receiving the "helper" data, the receiver try to reconstruct the secret key using the another feature set generated from the ECG signal. By the improved Juels and Sudan (IJS) algorithm, only the receiver that on the same body are able to reconstruct the secret key and decrypt the message. The ECG-IJS can secure the data transmission for WBANs, however, both the sender and receiver need to be coupled with an ECG sensor to sample ECG signals, which increases the hardware costs and brings in additional energy consumption. To address this problem, we further propose a channel information based authentication and encryption scheme (CIAE). Due to the symmetry channel, the received signal strength indicator (RSSI) measured at the sender and receiver are close enough to succeed the authentication.

Compared to the existing systems, the novelty of this work is in twofold: first, The proposed algorithms do not need prior key distribution or extra hardware. They use dynamic keys and work in a plug-n-play manner. The experimental results show that the proposed scheme is feasible to provide secure data wireless communications in a WBAN. The false acceptance rate (FAR) and false recognition rate (FRR) are also analyzed. Our studies show that the proposed schemes are a lightweight, work in a plug-n-play manner and energy efficient security solution for WBANs.

We addressed the inter-WBANs interference issues. Due to limited bands, WBANs are likely to have interference in real applications. The interference decline the signal to interference plus noise Ratio (SINR) and thereby cause throughput degradation and more packet loss, which leads to energy waste. We proposed a power game to mitigate the inter-network interference by adjusting the transmission powers. We applied the power game on both real and simulated social networks, the results demonstrated that proposed power game can efficiently mitigate the inter-network interference and increases the system's utility.

In summary, we have proposed ECG-IJS, an ECG-based authentication and encryption scheme, for WBANs applications. To remove the requirements of additional ECG sensors in ECG-IJS scheme, we further proposed CIAE, a channel information based authentication and encryption scheme for secure and private wireless transmissions in WBANs. After that, we also proposed a power control game to mitigate the inter-network interference among WBANs.

3.3 Concluding Remarks

Therefore, we conclude that a secure and intelligent architecture is required to support multiple wireless health applications.

References

Acock, A. C. (2005). Working with missing values. *J Marriage Fam*, 1012–1028.

Bao, S. D., Zhang, Y. T., & Shen, L. F. (2005). Physiological signal based entity authentication for body area sensor networks and mobile healthcare systems. *Engineering in Medicine and Biology Society, 2005. IEEE-EMBS 2005.* IEEE.

Bickel, P. J., & Freedman, D. A. (1981). Some asymptotic theory for the bootstrap. *Annals of Statistics*, 1196–1217.

Biel, L., Pettersson, O., Philipson, L., & Wide, P. (2001). Ecg analysis: a new approach in human identification. *IEEE Transactions on Instrumentation and Measurement*, 808–812.

Bollier, D., & Firestone, C. M. (2010). *The Promise and peril of big data.* Washington, DC, USA: Aspen Institute, Communications and Society Program.

Buck, S. F. (1960). A method of estimation of missing values in multivariate data suitable for use with an electronic computer. *Journal of the Royal Statistical Society. Series B, Statistical Methodology*, 302–306.

Chen, M., Gonzalez, S., Vasilakos, A., Cao, H., & Leung, V. C. (2011). Body area networks: A survey. *Mobile Networks and Applications*, 171–193.

Eysenbach, G. (2011). Consort-ehealth: Improving and standardizing evaluation reports of web-based and mobile health interventions. *Journal of Medical Internet Research*.

Fang, H., Espy, K. A., Rizzo, M. L., Stopp, C., Wiebe, S. A., & Stroup, W. W. (2009). Pattern recognition of longitudinal trial data with nonignorable missingness: An empirical case study. *International Journal of Information Technology & Decision Making*, 491–513.

Fang, H., Zhang, Z., Wang, C. J., Daneshmand, M., Wang, C., & Wang, H. (2015). A survey of big data research. *IEEE Networks*, 6–9.

Fang H et al. (n.d.). Retrieved from http://www.amstat.org/meetings/jsm/2014/onlineprogram/.

Little, R., & Rubin, D. (2014). *Statistical analysis with missing data.* Wiley.

Schafer, J. (1997). *Analysis of incomplete multivariate data.* CRC press.

Shao, J. (1993). Linear model selection by cross-validation. *Journal of the American Statistical Association*, 486–494.

Venkatasubramanian, K. K., Banerjee, A., & Gupta, S. K. (2008). Ekg-based key agreement in body sensor networks. *INFOCOM Workshops*, (pp. 1 –6).

Venkatasubramanian, K. K., Banerjee, A., & Gupta, S. K. S. (2010). PSKA: usable and secure key agreement scheme for body area networks. *Transactions on Information Technology*, 60–68.

Xie, X. L., & Beni, G. (1991). A validity measure for fuzzy clustering. *IEEE Transactions on Pattern Analysis and Machine Intelligence*, 841–847.

Zhang, Z., & Fang, H. (2016). Multiple-vs non-or single-imputation based fuzzy clustering for incomplete longitudinal behavioral intervention data. In *2016 IEEE first international conference on connected health: applications, systems and engineering technologies (CHASE)* (pp. 219–228). IEEE.

Zhang, Z., Wang, H., Vasilakos, A. V., & Fang, H. (2012). ECG-Cryptography and Authentication in Body Area Networks. *IEEE Transactions on Information Technology in Biomedicine*, 1070–1078.

Zhang, Z., Fang, H., & Wang, H. (2015). Visualization aided engagement pattern validation for big longitudinal web behavior intervention data. In *The 17th international Conference on E-health Networking, Application & Services. (IEEE Healthcom'15);.* Boston, USA: IEEE.

Chapter 4
Applications

4.1 Introduction

It is generally assumed that wearable technology is for personal use only, but it surely find its way in the enterprise world. It'll depend on the individuals and businesses to find out creative ways of using these wearables in improving their operational efficiencies, marketing, customer engagement and the way they do business. Here are few ways that wearable technologies could be used in business and commercial setups. Textiles are not only to protect/cover or skin, it shows self-expression, taste and personality of the wearer. It can also demonstrate socioeconomic status and cultural movements. Moreover, in the modern fashion world, wearable devices are highly relied on the beauty and aesthetic appeal. Recent advancement in wearable devices has extended the functionality of textile materials to "smart textile." Now the term smart textile referred as active or passive depends on the placement of actuators. If the actuator is embedded in textile, then it's active or passive in other cases. Smart textiles play a key role in our day to day life, including the fields of health monitoring, personal tracker, military, education, home appliances, transportation, gaming, entertainment and music. Reliable and continuous collection via wireless communications of patient vital signs such as blood pressure and flow, ECG (Electrocardiography), EEG (Electroencephalography), SPO2 is crucial for making real-time triage decisions. Multiple types of sensors collecting vital signs are connected to central control nodes (e.g., Smartphone and PDA) wirelessly. At a given time, a combination of multiple vital signs (biometric features) is unique to each patient. These features are important indicators to a clinician about patients' health status.

© The Author(s) 2016   39
H. Wang et al., *Wireless Health*, SpringerBriefs in Computer Science,
DOI 10.1007/978-3-319-47946-0_4

4.2 Wireless Health Applications

With the advancement of wireless technology, wireless devices can be used to reduce medical errors, increase medical care quality, improve the efficiency of caregivers, lessen the caregiver-lacking situation, and improve the comfort of patients. Although the technology has found ways into various fields, medical domain has very strict quality and assurance requirements, which causes many challenges that are faced when implementing and operating the systems. Although real-time patient monitoring field is not a new topic in wireless medical applications, researchers and industries are investing a lot of effort and money to it. These applications basically use biomedical sensors monitor the physiological signals of patients such as electro-cardiogram (ECG), blood oxygen level, blood pressures, blood glucose, coagulation, body weight, heart rate, EMG, ECG, oxygen saturation, etc. Home monitoring systems for chronic and elderly patients is rapidly growing up in quantity and quality. Using the system can reduce the hospital stay of patient and increase patient safety and mobility. The system collects periodic and continuous data and then transmits it to the centralized server. Patients' information is accessed by physicians remotely. These applications save large amount of time for doctors as well as patients. The doctors can monitor several patients simultaneously which is cannot be done by traditional monitoring, in which the patients are monitored directly by the doctors. The patients are no longer required to be present at the hospitals periodically.

Wireless sensor network can be applied to medical applications to build up databases for long-term clinical uses. It also can be used for emergency medical care and many other applications. The section presented the fields that wireless networks can contribute. The following part will identify challenge of deploying wireless networks based solutions in medical care.

With the advancement of wireless technology, wireless devices can be used to reduce medical errors, increase medical care quality, improve the efficiency of caregivers, lessen the caregiver-lacking situation, and improve the comfort of patients. Although the technology has found ways into various fields, medical domain has very strict quality and assurance requirements, which causes many challenges that are faced when implementing and operating the systems. Although real-time patient monitoring field is not a new topic in wireless medical applications, researchers and industries are investing a lot of effort and money to it. These applications basically use biomedical sensors monitor the physiological signals of patients such as electro-cardiogram (ECG), blood oxygen level, blood pressures, blood glucose, coagulation, body weight, heart rate, EMG, ECG, oxygen saturation, etc. Home monitoring systems for chronic and elderly patients is rapidly growing up in quantity and quality. Using the system can reduce the hospital stay of patient and increase patient safety and mobility. The system collects periodic and continuous data and then transmits it to the centralized server. Patients' information is accessed by physicians remotely. These applications save large amount of time for doctors as well as patients. The doctors can monitor several patients simultaneously which is cannot be done by traditional monitoring, in which the patients are monitored directly by the doctors. The patients may be no longer required to be present at the hospitals periodically.

- **Textile Sensor**

Textiles are not only to protect/cover or skin, it shows self-expression, taste and personality of the wearer. It can also demonstrate socio-economic status and cultural movements. Moreover, in the modern fashion world, textiles are highly relied on the beauty and aesthetic appeal. Recent advancement in wearable devices has extended the functionality of textile materials to "smart textile." Now the term smart textile referred as active or passive depends on the placement of actuators. If the actuator is embedded in textile, then it's active or passive in other cases. Smart textiles play a key role in our day to day life, including the fields of health monitoring, personal tracker, military, education, home appliances, transportation, gaming, entertainment and music. Table 4.1 shows the fundamental applications of smart/intelligent textiles.

- **Sports**

Wearing smart textiles in the sports sector have certainly improved their performance, personal comfort and awareness. It also fueled many research in smart textile industry, for example, breathable textile and moisture management textile (Bello, Darling, & Lipoma, 2011). New invention on smart textile has allowed to control the body temperature using phase change technology, the working principle is to absorb the surplus heat and release it when needed. The recent advancement in textile material it is possible to sense the instantaneous biological condition and biochemical status of athletes. The piezo-electric sensor stitched into textile material can help to kinematic analysis, which may be able to correct posture, enhance movements and reduce injuries. Moreover, wearable textile sensors are always active for continuous monitoring and provide real time vital

Table 4.1 Application of different wearable sensor technology

Health monitoring	Blood pressure, patches, heart rate monitoring, ECG monitoring, hearing aids, visual aids, remote drug delivery, emergency help, air filters, healing devices, antibiotic, insulin injection, glucose check, sleep apnea
Electronics and computers	Computer and TV screens, games, computer hardware, solar cell, motion detector, gaming console
Fitness tracker	Personal tracker, activity monitoring, calorie counter, posture tracking
	Active walking, strain resistant cloths, sleep sensor, smart glass, smart cloths
Military	Hand-worn terminals, head-up display, smart clothing, smart glass, remote medic, personal tracking device
Industrial	Hand-worn devices, smart clothing, finger tracking, gesture based devices
Food	Temperature control, germproof refrigerator, calorie counter

information to track performance. Smart training socks can also be categorized as wearable sensors, this consists of RFID tag, wireless module, motion sensor and accelerometer. Additionally, textile sensors can be used as a personal activity tracker such as calorie consumption, HRV and quality of sleep. Future of smart textile may be involving chemical sensors embedded in clothes where the information can be extracted from sweat analysis.

- **Industrial Applications**

In industries, many workers need one or two hands to complete the tasks, and as well as they have to keep up clear vision. Wearable textile has different advantages depending on the industrial need. As wearable sensors offer portability, flexibility and easy to use, industries have started to adopt this trend. Smart textiles with head mounted display and hands-free option can provide solutions for many type industries. We have mentioned before, the first industry to adopt wearable textile was The Boeing Company. In 2014, Mercedes-Benz presented pebble smart watch where a user can check on fuel level, location and door lock. The tiny watch can also alert before any incoming calls, emails, and texts, which makes it a remote display of your smart phone. From behind the when, user can as well monitor road accident, construction and parked vehicles. It also comes with three customizable buttons to access media, auto-routing, voice activation and remote start.

- **Biomedical Applications**

Location and navigation based application is always the basic requirement of the many sensor networks. For continuous and long-term monitoring of physiological information can be fulfilled but smart textile. Commercially available devices offer long-term monitoring of heart rate, ECG, oxygen, respiration and body temperature. Many of the applications have been developed based on textile sensors, such as fall detection, heart rate variability (HRV) and pulse rate. Textile sensors can also be used for wireless health monitoring and measure—the how and—the what of the user. In the medical science wearable sensor has achieved more success than any other field. An example can be given by textile sensor is remote insulin level monitoring. Like, for a diabetic patient rather than injecting insulin all the time, smart textile can be used to provide insulin when the insulin level gets lower than the threshold. In addition, it can reduce the visiting frequency of a patient, and also minor injuries/illness can be operated from a remote location. Smart textile promotes the prevention health care, because current focuses are moving from treatment to prevention.

The Remote Monitoring System (RMS) was developed at Mayo Clinic to support and monitor the cardiac patient. There is a commercially available textile based wearable sensor, for example, BodyTel and BioMan t-shirt. A new concept in healthcare monitoring is emerging through the ground-breaking smart and intelligent sensor to be worn without any physical discomfort. WEALTHY and MyHeart is two EU funded projects. WEALTHY system will be consisted of full server backup of the decision making system integrated with smart sensors, wireless module and highly scalable computing techniques. MyHeart is one of the biggest health care research projects funded by the European Union. The project first came up with the heart failure management system, which can predict early heart failure.

Previously, textile fabrics were only used for fashion, appearance, comfort and protection; however, smart textile can extend the health monitoring system to a modern level by utilizing touch, chemical, and pressure sensors. Adding nanotechnology to smart textile can open a whole new generation of telemedicine and health care application.

- **Military Applications**

Wearable textile sensors can be used to identify dangerous chemicals and biological weapons. The most advantage of using smart textiles instead of current chemical sensor is that it can detect very low concentration of changes. For critical conditions and hazardous situations, soldiers may need further help for navigation and access to tactical information. Enhance version of smart textiles with more capabilities can assist law enforce agencies and defense forces. Recent researches have shown that smart textile can detect environmental changes such as toxic gas. This can also help soldiers to identify between a friendly and hostile zone instantaneously. Wearable sensor has to be very close to the targeted area and must collide with physically. Another application is medics can perform triages remotely and rapidly.

- **Environmental Applications**

In the environment, the applications for embedded textile sensors are many. Detection of the chemical contaminates in the tree is one of the recent advancement of the nanosensors integrated into woven fabrics. Nanotechnology can be used to improve our collection of measurement at low-cost and for a longer period of time. Chemical nanosensors can be used to detect harmful compounds in tree, herbs and bushes, which usually released chemicals in the air.

- **Fashion**

No matter how and where we put the sensor on clothing, it has to be fashionable. The fashion and sensor designers will find a way to use their creativity and make the proper functional system without hampering the appearance, giving new and stunning effects. With technological enhancement, sensors are getting miniaturized and systems are becoming unnoticeable. Already there are switches available in the market as smart textile t-shirt. Light emitting textiles are finding its way to emerge in future smart garments.

- **Movement and Finger Tracking**

This may be implemented by using smart textile. Computer will recognize/track every movement of the wearer; this can be used for gaming, controlling multiple computers or designing tools.

4.3 The Trends of Wearable Technologies

4.3.1 Current Technology Literature and Wearable Computing

Employee Wellness: To monitor employee's health condition as a part wellness program, companies can deploy wearable devices. This data can be tied into health insurance policy premiums or other incentive programs to reduce health care costs.

Demonstrations, training, troubleshooting: Virtual reality headsets like Oculus Rifts can be utilized for training and demonstrate what exactly one is seeing in real-time. For technical troubleshooting augmented reality can perform a guide to users how and what to do. This also has merits in multiple industries, like hospitality, real estate, advertising, healthcare, mechanical, construction, etc.

Travel: Wearable devices, like Google Glass, can help to traveler and business person to directly access information like maps, direction and weather conditions using their smartphones.

Sports and Entertainment: Smart textiles and wearable cameras can improve the performance of the game, it can be used by sportsmen, athletes or stage performers, which can capture their movements, metrics and experiences that can be shared with their fans. Wearing smart textiles in the sports sector have certainly improved their performance, personal comfort and awareness. It also fueled many research in smart textile industry, for example, breathable textile and moisture management textile. New invention on smart textile has allowed to control the body temperature using phase change technology, the working principle is to absorb the surplus heat and release it when needed. The recent advancement in textile material it is possible to sense the instantaneous biological condition and biochemical status of athletes. The piezoelectric sensor stitched into a textile material can help to kinematic analysis, which may be able to correct posture, enhance movements and reduce injuries. Moreover, wearable textile sensors are always active for continuous monitoring and provide real time vital information to track performance. Smart training socks can also be categorized as wearable sensors, which consist of RFID tag, wireless module, motion sensor and accelerometer. Additionally, textile sensors can be used as a personal activity tracker such as calorie consumption, HRV and quality of sleep. Future of smart textile may be involving chemical sensors embedded in clothes where the information can be extracted from sweat analysis.

Advertising: Wearable devices are enabling more areas for business to connect mass people. This also adds value and revenues to advertise industries.

Shopping: Wearable technology will give organization to get a better understating of consumer behavior, and start a new level of interconnected services. Walmart, Amazon and all the big retailers can utilize this information to set their targeted customers.

Shipping and Logistics: Fitness bands can play an important role in the shipping industries. For example, Tesco has provided a wristband to employees to mark the good has been delivered on time, eliminating the need to mark clipboards and giving mangers estimated completion times.

Police, traffic and security: Wearable technology can play a key role for police, security and traffic officials. For instance, Google Glass or smart camera can capture all the details of daily activities around police officials, can take evidence of traffic violators, accidents or unexpected incidents. A smart watch can be useful for alerting of accidents or sending alert signals

Emergency Workers: A smartwatch or fitness band might help organizations to monitor their workers health, it can notify medical personnel in case of emergency. Worker health information could be useful for health insurance companies, hence reduce health care cost.

Sales and Marketing: This wearable device will create new opportunities for sales and marketing, which includes smarter and fastest way to access big data. Making a robust customer data storage and manipulation, it will help for sudden decision making. Sales professionals can get access to CRM or prospect/client information on the go. Augmented reality devices can be used in giving product demonstrations.

4.3.2 Future IoT for Healthcare

(a) **Nano Sensors**:

Nanotechnology has enabled us to manufacture and design systems in the scale of nanometer level. This also exhibits different properties of material which cannot be even displayed at the microscopic level. The goal of this technology is to create miniature devices with functionality with special attributes. There are two kinds of nano-material, one is intentionally produced nano-materials and the other is just naturally made. By the characteristics of nanotechnology, it does not include unintentionally produced nano-materials, for example, diesel exhaust particle or other byproducts. However, there is a subdivision of intentionally produced nano-materials. For example, a nano-sensor with silver nano-particle works as artificial skin. It is very sensitive to pressure or any kind of deformation.

Nanotechnology has a great potential for creating new systems and materials with special characteristics. Such as improved efficiency, increased thermal and electrical conductivity and increased robustness of the systems, these all can be done with nanotechnology. In addition, of commercial products, nanotechnology has great effect on the environment too. A nano size cerium oxide has been manufactured to reduce the diesel emissions in the soil. Nano-senors can be used to track and detect toxicities in soil and water. So, there are thousands of applications yet to discover as we get more knowledge on nanotechnology. One of the first application of nanotechnology is nano-sensors. A nano-sensor does not have to be on the scale of nanometers rather is using the special property of the nano-particles to send and detect the information in nano scale. Like, nano-sensors can detect and measure concentrations of chemical compounds as low as one part per billion (Daniel et al., n.d.). For intra communication between two nano-sensors will increase the complexity as well as the applications. To cover a large area with nano-sensors we need a solid network between them. Current nano-sensors need excitation and measurement from external method to operate. However, introducing wireless communication will surely eliminate these requirements. In Wakamiya (2016), they have discussed thoroughly about nano communications and sensors. Researchers and scientists are still experimenting on nano-sensor based applications such as medical science, agriculture, cosmetics, food and paint. In medical science, there is a tool to synthesize cancer treatment more efficiently. Using nanotechnology as a carrier of medicine has significant improvement in the ordinary drug treatment. Additionally, it reduces the toxicity and increase the efficiency. Even in the agriculture field nano-composites can be used to eliminate weeds and improve the fertilization of the soil. However, there is not enough information to assess environmental exposure to manufactured nano-materials. Apart from all the benefits of nanotechnology possess, we need to understand the effects of human life and ecosystems.

(b) **Non-contact Sensor**:

A non-contact monitoring system is sensing information without physical contact with the subject. Many researches have been done recently to maximize the accuracy at low cost. The variety of non-contact sensors regarding medical purposes which span from heart rate to acoustic sensors creates a set of technical requirements with a wide variation in terms of expected performance metrics, as throughput or delay, therefore good architectures and protocols are needed. Different sensors can be used depending on the desired application. Generally, optical, electromagnetic, acoustic, and pneumatic procedures can be utilized to acknowledge non-contact estimation of physiological amounts. The obtained vital information about human body can be observed either via a wireless or a wired link like patches or implanted sensors which may result distress to the patient. Hence, the advantages of non-contact sensor is they do not discomfort to the patient usual activity, whereas with the wearable sensors user have to use patches or inject the sensors. Which can cause injuries or bruises to a patient.

There has been a lot of work regarding non-contact health monitoring in the previous years. In this section different type's method has depicted to describe the system's functionality and components. However, this should not be perceived as the standard system design, as many systems may adopt significantly varying architectural or functional approaches. In Cauwenberghs (2010), they have introduced a new method to monitor different method for monitoring respiration signal and heart rate. The aim of the paper was to provide a contactless microwave sensor, allowing continual remote monitoring of the heartbeat and respiratory rates. This work provided a comparative study to signal detection of a heartbeat, considering different frequencies and transmission powers. They have varied the frequency a power level of the system to compare and analyze the difference between the outputs of the system. They have used Vector Network analyzer and two horn antenna to extract the vital information's. Also, the calculated the phase difference between input and output, and concluded that as the phase variation increases the sensitivity of the small displacement frequency increases, hence improve the accuracy for tiny displacement. However, with increasing frequency the power level increase so the power level has to be in certain level so that it does effect the user. In addition, of the previous method a radar-based health monitoring system, enabling non-invasive fall detection and tag-less localization in the home environment has been presented and discussed in Torkestani, Julien-Vergonjanne, and Cances (2010). They depicted a success rate of 94.3 % in distinguishing fall events from normal movements and a good detection of the target's absolute distance. The detection of falls together with tag less indoor localization can be made contactless by adopting radar techniques. The radar is used to transmit an RF signal to a person and to receive the reflected echo, on the basis of which the person's speed and absolute distance can be extracted. It consists of a sensor, combining radar sensing and Zigbee wireless communications, and microcontroller capabilities, and of a Zigbee equipped base station for data processing. But, backscattering and crosstalk effects have to be in minimum level because the backscattering within the frequency band where the sensor is used to locate the target and determine its speed must be strongly reduced to enable maximum forward power towards the target. If the system is unable to reduce the backscattering will obviously limit the forward transmit power, resulting in a weak reflection from the target, and in a waste of energy. Another challenge was to get the semispherical radiation pattern as they had to cover the whole room. So to eliminate this problem they reduce the length between the sensor and the patient. Additionally used multiple antenna for localization. The heart rate can be measured by extracting fluctuation of human eyes. Researches designed a system where they can observe the heart rate variability (HRV) with the help of a popular movement of the patient. The architecture is to track the papillary with imaging and an integral-differential algorithm by segmenting the pupiliris boundary. They estimated HRV from the relative distribution of energy in the low frequency (0.04–0.15 Hz) and high frequency (0.15–0.4 Hz) bands of the power spectrum of the time series of popular fluctuations. And then they validated the method under a range of breathing conditions and under different illumination levels. The whole process as follows, first, the eye has to be tracked and then with image processing the corneal reflection was removed. After detecting the pupil-iris boundary using an integral-differential operator, which allows us to compute the pupil diameter, the system was used to monitor fluctuations in pupil diameter to extract an index of HRV. The problem with that system is to track the pupil and then remove the corneal reflection due to occlusion by the eyelids and eyelashes, corneal reflections, the color of the eye, imaging angle, etc. To overcome this method they have used the conventional method that was introduced that is robust to occlusions caused by the upper and lower eyelids. The algorithm assumes the pupil and iris have circular geometry, and uses an integral-differential operator to locate the boundaries between them. The pulse radar system works by sending short electromagnetic pulses and receiving the echoes reflected by the target. The time delay between the transmitted pulse and received echo is given by the time of flight of the pulse (round trip from transmitter to receiver) which is therefore proportional to the distance from the target to the radar. With the same methodology vital parameters of the human body have been deployed. The field operational tests demonstrate that the UWB radar sensor detects the respiratory rate of person under test (adult and baby) associated with sub-centimeter chest movements, allowing the continuous-time non-invasive monitoring of hospital patients and other people at risk of obstructive apneas such as babies in cot beds, or other respiratory diseases. Additionally, with respect to continuous wave (CW) radars, UWB radar transceivers present a lower circuit complexity since no frequency conversions are required, leading to lower power consumption for longer battery autonomy. The complexity arises when the subject is moving, in a static position the signal at the output of the Integrator is pretty much constant. But if the target is moving, the movement causes a time-varying between the local replica and the echo amplified by the network analyzer. Therefore, the multiplier provides an output pulse that may be positive, negative or zero, depending on the caused by the time-varying distance between radar and target and due to the target movements around its quiescent position.

Example of Non-contact sensor: The basic concept of ECG electrodes was derived from the electro-chemicals from the human body generated by oxidation and reduction reactions between a metal plate and human skin. The current system is a perfect example of this description. A wet Ag/AgCl electrode contains a half-cell potential, creating two sets of parallel series resistance as shown in Fig. 4.1. But for non-contact capacitive electrodes, the electrochemical circuit is much different than that were seen for gel electrodes. Usually, non-contact sensor coupling between skin and conductor plate creates a series combination of a parallel RC

Fig. 4.1 Coupling factor of skin-electrode for (*left*) wet Ag/AgCl electrodes and (*right*) Non-contact electrodes. RG = Gel Resistance, CG = Capacitance Resistance, RSC and CSC the resistance and capacitance of the Stratum Comeum respectively, CGAP = Capacitance due to air gap, RC = Cotton Resistance and CC = Cotton Capacitance (Mobile Biopotential Monitoring Suite, University of California, San Diego)

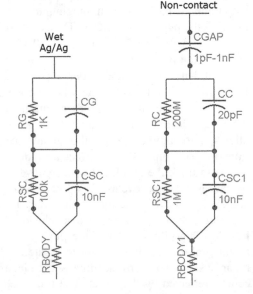

circuit and a capacitance in series due to the gap between electrodes and human skin. One of the two sets of RC circuit dominates the coupling factor and represented as a single component. Furthermore, both resistance and capacitance in non-contact electrodes are equally important. However, the general norm to have a high conductance or low resistance in the electrodes can be misleading in certain cases. To reduce the grounding effect, we have used virtual ground. The ECG signal is then routed through multiple stages of amplification and filtration. After analog to digital conversion, it can be transmitted through a wireless node to any kind of mobile, computer, and personal server or to a medical doctor.

Compared to conventional wet electrodes, capacitive-based electrode should be a good alternative to provide no discomfort while measures vital information. The current system uses a resistive method while the capacitive method is carried using a conductor and an insulator in between the skin and the electrode. Based on different research, there are some insulators which can be used in capacitive-based ECG sensors, such as silicon dioxide, pyre varnish, and barium titanate. However, in our experiments, we have used cotton as insulation. One drawback of capacitive-based electrodes is signals are not as strong as gel-based electrodes due to the high impedance of human skin and the fact that our bodies work as an antenna which affects noise in the signal. The significant factor of a capacitive-coupled ECG system is that even with a little displacement between the electrode and skin, there will be a change in the coupling capacitance; hence, the signal will be distorted by motion (Fig. 4.2).

Figure 4.3 depicts the design of a portable health monitoring bed for infants. The size of the bed is 120 cm × 200 cm, and four load cells have been installed between the frame and the surface of the bed. These load cells are connected in Wheatstone bridge configuration, the output resistance changes with the change of the forces. The output of the sensors is connected to the dedicated analog front end. The analog front end consists of multiple filters and amplifiers. The purpose of the AFE is to extract, amplify, and filter small bio-potential signal in the presence of different noise sources. For high input impedance, a buffer circuit is added to the front end, analog circuit and proper shielding was used to reduce the

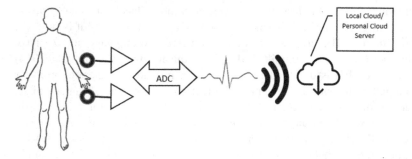

Fig. 4.2 Basic architecture of wireless BSN. The system consists of an EPIC sensor with proposed analog signal and low power wireless module

Fig. 4.3 Schematic diagram
of measuring BCG signal of a
healthy human heart

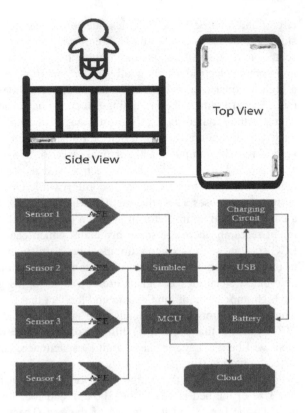

electromagnetic interference. The front end circuit starts with a buffer amplifier LMP7701 which helps to improve the input impedance and bootstraps the biasing network. The output signal is connected to AD8221, an ultra-high input impedance instrumental amplifier. This provides the differential gain and drives the common line. The multiple HPF and LPF have been used to reduce the low and high frequency components. The analog circuit is designed for optimal performance with very low power consumption. A 60 Hz notch filter is also used to remove baseline fluctuation noises. Wireless microprocessor Simblee has been used to process the data coming from AFE. It is suitable for IoT applications, and it is only 7 mm × 10 mm in size. The firmware was based on Arduino language and we have used Arduino 1.6.1 IDE to compile and upload the firmware (Koo et al., 2014). The unique algorithm is designed to save power; instead of transmitting all the raw data together, it sends a fragment of the full data. That is an advantage of scalable model. Additionally, it has 512 kB memory to store the data for later acquisition or other purposes. To visualize the analog signal, a graphical user interface is used, which is developed in Processing software. It also includes the software level manipulation too, but at a minor level, so that we can see the real time simulation.

4.4 Concluding Remarks

Location and navigation based applications are always the basic requirement of the many sensor networks. Continuous and long-term monitoring of physiological information can be fulfilled by wearable technology. Commercially available devices offer long-term monitoring of heart rate, ECG, oxygen, respiration and body temperature. Many of the applications have been developed based on textile sensors, such as fall detection, heart rate variability (HRV) and pulse rate. Textile sensors can also be used for wireless health monitoring and measure—the how and—the what of the user. In the medical science wearable sensor has achieved more success than any other field. An example can be given by textile sensor is remote insulin level monitoring. Like, for a diabetic patient rather than injecting insulin all the time, smart textile can be used to provide insulin when the insulin level gets lower than the threshold. In addition, it can reduce the visiting frequency of a patient, and also minor injuries/illness can be operated from a remote location. Smart textile promotes the prevention and healthcare, while current focuses are moving from treatment to prevention.

The Remote Monitoring System (RMS) was developed at Mayo Clinic to support and monitor the cardiac patient. There is a commercially available textile based wearable sensor. For example, BodyTel and BioMan T-shirt. A new concept in healthcare monitoring is emerging through the groundbreaking smart and intelligent sensor to be worn without any physical discomfort. WEALTHY and MyHeart is two EU funded projects. WEALTHY system will be consisted of full server backup of the decision making system integrated with smart sensors, wireless module and highly scalable computing techniques. MyHeart is one of the biggest health care research projects funded by the European Union. The project first came up with the heart failure management system, which can predict early heart failure. Previously, textile fabrics were only used for fashion, appearance, comfort and protection; however, smart textile can extend the health monitoring system to a modern level by utilizing touch, chemical, and pressure sensors. Adding nanotechnology to smart textile can open a whole new generation of telemedicine and health care application.

References

Bello, J. P., Darling, C. J., & Lipoma T. S. (2011). A sleep diagnostics shirt employing respiratory patterns through chest expansion. *The international conference on design of medical devices*. Minneapolis, MN, USA.

Cauwenberghs, Y. M. (2010). Wireless non-contact EEG/ECG electrodes for body sensor networks. *Body Sensor Networks (BSN)-2010*. Singapore: IEEE.

Daniel, S., Rao, T. P., Rao, K. S., Rani, S. U., Naidu, G. R. K., Lee, H. Y., ... & Kawai, T. (n.d.). A review of DNA functionalized/grafted carbon nanotubes and their characterization. *Sensors and Actuators B: Chemical*, 672–682.

Koo, H. R., Lee, Y. J., Gi, S., Khang, S., Lee, J. H., Lee, J. H., … & Lee, J. W. (2014). The effect of textile-based inductive coil sensor positions for heart rate monitoring. *Journal of Medical System*.

Torkestani, S. S., Julien-Vergonjanne, A., & Cances, J. P. (2010). Mobile healthcare monitoring in hospital based on diffuse optical wireless technology. In *IEEE 21st international symposium on personal indoor and mobile radio communications (PIMRC)* (pp. 1055–1059). IEEE.

Wakamiya, F. P. (2016). Low-complexity nanosensor networking through spike-encoded signaling. *IEEE Internet of Things Journal*, 49–58.

Chapter 5
Conclusion and Future Directions

The development of wireless technologies such as 5G, mobile devices, sensors, and robots have shaped our life in multiple aspects. New Wireless health and system technologies aim to enabling the ubiquitous healthcare anytime and anywhere to improve health and wellbeing. At the same time, wireless health systems and computer technologies are capable of doing real-time and remote monitoring at a home, community, city, or medical hospital. We believe that these health technologies not only enable preventive care and early-detection, but also significantly reduce the healthcare cost. This book talks about the opportunities advances of wireless health, and shares our studies learned from several wireless health projects. With further advances of sensing, communications, and intelligent techniques, more and more wireless health applications will grow in the market, serving the purpose of saving people's lives and improving the well beings.

© The Author(s) 2016
H. Wang et al., *Wireless Health*, SpringerBriefs in Computer Science,
DOI 10.1007/978-3-319-47946-0_5

Printed in the United States
By Bookmasters